In the middle of a party full of drugged teenagers, one boy lay unconscious on the floor . . .

"Are you okay?" I yelled but the boy didn't move. "Wake up. Wake up!" I took the knuckle of my index finger and ground it into the boy's breastbone. There was no reaction.

I looked at the boy who had beckoned us over. "What happened?"

"I don't know," he replied. "He just went out."

"What is he on?"

"Nothing," he answered defensively . . .

Suddenly, the boy's eyes flew open and he shot up into a sitting position. Wild-eyed, he looked down at his feet, then turned his dilated pupils toward me.

"You stole my shoes," he shrieked, his eyes boring into mine, "and I'm going to kill you!" At that moment, I was sure he could . . .

RESCUE ALERT

JOAN E. LLOYD & EDWIN B. HERMAN

BERKLEY BOOKS, NEW YORK

RESCUE ALERT

A Berkley Book / published by arrangement with
the authors

PRINTING HISTORY
Berkley edition / January 1994

For information address: The Berkley Publishing Group,
200 Madison Avenue, New York, New York 10016.

ISBN: 0-425-14052-0

BERKLEY®
Berkley Books are published by The Berkley Publishing Group,
200 Madison Avenue, New York, New York 10016.
BERKLEY and the "B" design
are trademarks belonging to Berkley Publishing Corporation.

PRINTED IN THE UNITED STATES OF AMERICA

10 9 8 7 6 5 4 3 2 1

ACKNOWLEDGMENTS

We would like to thank all the past and present members of the "Fairfax" Volunteer Ambulance Corps with whom we have ridden over the years. We would also like to thank the members of other local ambulance corps and rescue squads with whom we have taken calls. We would also like to acknowledge the invaluable assistance we have gotten over the years from the members of the "Fairfax" Police Department, the "Fairfax" Fire Department, and so many others.

And we would like to thank all of those who, having heard that we were writing a book, were kind enough to share their experiences with us.

And, "Greg," thanks for parting with your recipes.

In ambulance work, we see the best and the worst. When we save a life or give comfort to an ill or injured person, it is a phenomenal high. When we lose a patient or witness the results of a senseless act that ends in needless suffering or death, we ourselves often become angry or sad.

We would like to dedicate this book to Arielle and Davida Herman, and Elizabeth and Judy Lloyd. Davida and Judy have ridden with us, Arielle and Judy have helped with this manuscript, and all four of our children have shared the joy and have given us help and support for the pain.

Thanks.

ONE

FIFTY-YEAR-OLD CHARLIE SHAY had gone to the A&P with his wife, June, to do the weekly marketing. He spent much of the trip through the aisles backseat driving each of his wife's purchases and dipping into an open box of chocolate chip cookies. June stopped at the salad bar and filled a clear plastic container with lettuce, tomatoes, green peppers, and broccoli, despite Charlie's complaints that he hated broccoli almost as much as George Bush did.

As June pushed the cart toward the soda aisle, Charlie reached under the clear plastic cover of the salad bar, grabbed a pickle out of the pickle juice, took a bite, and chewed noisily.

As the Shays proceeded toward the back of the store, a middle-aged man in an A&P employees' jacket entered the aisle from the other end pushing a hand truck filled with cases of soda. Charlie, afraid that the employee would catch him with his stolen pickle, shoved the entire thing into his mouth. It stuck in his throat.

With an irritated expression on his face, Charlie tried to cough, but the pickle wouldn't budge. He tried to draw in another gulp of air to again attempt to cough out the offending object. With the pickle wedged tightly in his airway, he couldn't inhale and therefore he couldn't cough, or speak, or breathe. Frantically, Charlie grabbed his wife's arm and gestured so she would understand that he was choking. As his lips moved silently, June suddenly understood and started to scream. "Help! Help him! I think he's choking."

While a young employee ran to call an ambulance, shoppers flocked to the soda aisle.

"Pound him on the back!"

"Get him some water!"

"Someone grab him and do that choking thing. I saw it on TV."

June whirled around. "Does anyone know how to do that hug thing? You've got to help him."

But no one knew how to do the Heimlich maneuver. The more the man struggled to breathe, the tighter the pickle lodged in his throat.

I had stopped at headquarters to pick up whatever was in my corps mailbox when the claxon blasted its strident tones.

"Fairfax Police to Fairfax Ambulance."

Heather Franks leapt from her chair in the headquarters kitchen and pressed the transmit button on the microphone. "Fairfax Ambulance on, go ahead."

"The ambulance is needed at the A&P in town for a person choking."

I stuck my head into the kitchen. "Need another?" I said, not knowing who was on duty.

"Yeah," said Sam Middleton, the other member on duty. Sam was a relatively new member of the Fairfax Volunteer Ambulance Corps who was still taking his EMT course. He was a professional firefighter and was the driver today. I knew that Heather was on her first call since getting her certification as an EMT-D, an emergency medical technician with added training in defibrillation.

"10–4, Fairfax Police, 45–01 is responding."

"The caller seems to think that the victim isn't breathing," the police dispatcher said. "Expedite."

"Joan," Heather said to me, "would you crew chief this one?"

"I'll back you up if you want to take it."

"I'd rather you take over. I don't feel ready for this just yet."

I nodded, then leaned over and keyed the mike. "Page out for one more member," I said to the police dispatcher, "and have him respond directly to the scene."

"10–4. FPD clear."

Sam jumped into the driver's seat and I rode shotgun, in the passenger seat. When Sam had pulled the rig clear of the giant garage door, Heather closed it and climbed into the back of the ambulance. Lights flashing and siren screaming, the vehicle sped across town. From the rig radio I could hear the sounds of our pager tones as the police tried to get us more manpower.

Although I knew that Sam and Heather would eventually become good EMTs, they were both new and inexperienced. Despite several requests for extra manpower, however, no one else had called in. We would have to make do. We pulled up in front of the supermarket, and Sam and I jumped out.

"I'll bring the stretcher," Heather said as Sam grabbed the crash bag. "You two go ahead."

Together, Sam and I ran through the wide automatic doors. We looked around the store, but at first we couldn't locate the victim.

"This way," a breathless employee said as he ran up and gestured wildly toward the rear of the store, "by the sodas." Led by the young A&P clerk, we ran across the front of the store and turned down the soda aisle. As I loped toward the gathered crowd, I saw two police officers running from the other direction. Most of the Fairfax Police officers are CPR certified so I knew that I could use one of them if I needed extra hands.

The crowd surrounded the supine figure of a man in his fifties. His eyes were closed and his color was not encouraging. His skin was pale and his lips had a bluish tinge. As I knelt next to him I could see the store manager restraining the man's tiny wife. She screamed, "He's not dead. He can't die. Charlie, you've got to breathe!"

"Sir," I yelled, shaking the man's shoulder. "Sir, can you hear me?" I got no reaction.

I hyperextended the man's neck to try to provide an airway, and I asked, "Any idea what happened?"

"He just keeled over!" his wife screamed. "I think he strangled on something."

I listened to hear whether any air was passing through Charlie's mouth while I pressed my fingers against the side of his neck, feeling for his carotid artery. He was not breathing, but I could feel a weak, thready pulse.

"No one could do that choking thing," a voice intoned. "Then he just crumpled to the floor."

As I opened the man's mouth, I could see about an inch of the end of what looked like a pickle projecting from his throat. I quickly pulled on a latex glove, reached into his mouth, grasped the end of the object, and pulled. The end was slippery and tapering and it slid through my gloved fingers. After a few attempts, I decided to try to give a breath around the object.

"What's his name?" I asked.

"Charlie. Charlie Shay," his wife said.

As I took my CPR mask and used Charlie's jawbone to lift his lower jaw, I said, "Stay with us, Charlie. We're taking good care of you." I hoped he could hear me.

I pressed Charlie's face against the mask so that it would seal over his mouth and nose, and attempted to blow air into his lungs. I couldn't get air past the object.

Impatiently, I yanked off my glove, pushed the mask aside and again reached into the man's mouth. I used my fingernails to try to skewer the pickle, but although I could get a little better grip, I still couldn't dislodge it.

"Clear away," I said as I slipped into the CPR instructor's equivalent of autopilot. "I need room." The crowd moved back, and I crawled around the patient and straddled his thighs. I placed the heel of one hand on his lower abdomen, put my other hand on top, and gave him eight abdominal thrusts.

No success.

I scrambled around to the patient's head and tried again to dislodge the pickle. It wouldn't move. I tried again to give a breath.

Nothing.

The patient was slipping deeper and deeper into unconsciousness, which meant that his muscles were relaxing more and more. Although his condition was worsening, this might now make it easier to dislodge the pickle. There was still a chance.

Heather and another policeman arrived with the stretcher. We quickly lifted our patient onto the stretcher while Sam positioned a special CPR board under his head. The board served two purposes; it would keep his neck hyperextended so that his airway would remain open, and it would give us a hard surface to work on if we began CPR. CPR would be useless, however, until we could get air into Charlie's lungs.

"Don't roll yet," I said as they began to pull the stretcher toward the door. "Let me give it one more try." I straddled the stretcher, administered another series of abdominal thrusts and attempted to remove the pickle from the man's airway. I hoped that the movement of his body might have dislodged it, but the object still didn't budge. The area around the man's lips was blue, and I knew that if I felt for a carotid pulse again there would be none.

Marge Talbot, a longtime corps member, handed me the bag-valve-mask attached to an oxygen tank. "When did you get here?" I asked her. I had been so focused on trying to ventilate my patient that I had not noticed her arrival.

"A few minutes ago. I was working at home today, and as soon as I reached a stopping-off place in the audit I was running, I came right over."

"Great. I'm glad to see you." I pressed the mask over the man's mouth and nose and squeezed the bag. It was always possible that just enough air was getting into his lungs to keep his brain supplied with oxygen.

Quickly, we rolled the stretcher to the rig and loaded it into the back. Heather, Marge, and I scrambled into the back and Sam got into the cab to drive.

As the ambulance started toward the hospital, code 3, lights and siren, Heather used the onboard radio and called the hospital. "Fairfax ambulance 45–01 to Fairfax emergency room."

"Fairfax hospital on. Go ahead 45–01."

"Be advised that we're en route to your location with a man of undetermined age with an obstructed airway. Unable to ventilate at this time. Our ETA is five minutes."

The rig turned on to route 10, and I pulled on the pickle for what seemed like the hundredth time. Suddenly I felt it shift, slip, and come loose. Triumphantly, I pulled it from the man's mouth. "I got it!" I called. I fitted the mask over his mouth and nose, lifted his jaw, and squeezed the bag. I saw his chest rise. "Yeah," I yelled. Finally, he had a clear airway and oxygen was getting into his lungs. I quickly squeezed again and watched oxygen again fill his lungs.

I pulled the mask away, leaned down, and placed my ear close to Charlie's mouth. I gently placed my fingers on his carotid pulse. I quickly determined that, although he now had an airway, he had no pulse and wasn't breathing on his own. "No pulse or breathing," I said as I slipped an oral airway into his mouth to keep his tongue from obstructing his now-clear airway. "I'll hold the mask and Marge can squeeze the bag. Heather, can you do compressions?"

"Sure." Heather quickly located the compression site in the middle of the man's sternum. All the way to the hospital, I held the CPR mask sealed against the man's face while Marge squeezed the bag in rhythm with Heather's compressions. Periodically, I rechecked Charlie's vitals, but he still had neither breathing nor pulse.

At the hospital, as we pulled the stretcher out of the back of the rig, I saw the man's wife arrive in a police car. As we pushed the stretcher and continued CPR, the police kept the hysterical woman in the car, out of our way.

I sometimes think of the strange dichotomy we feel. People who work in emergency medical services develop strong defenses against the pain, suffering, and death that have become a part of our lives. It's not that we don't care about the people we treat; if we didn't care we wouldn't risk so much to save them. But if we stopped and thought about who the person was, whose husband he was, or who called him Daddy, the emotional toll when a patient didn't recover would be devastating.

In the beginning, we make a conscious effort to separate ourselves from our patients, but somewhere along the way, it becomes second nature. It's a fine line we walk, though, because the defensive wall must not be too thick. The psychological first aid we administer to our patients and their loved ones is, at times, more critical than the medical aid. Each patient is experiencing his own personal crisis and his need for emotional support must not be ignored. So we walk the line between giving effective psychological care to our patients and retaining our own emotional defenses.

We wheeled the man through the ER doors. The emergency room doors would prevent his wife from accompanying him. We transferred him to the gurney, and I told the triage nurse, "His airway was completely obstructed with a piece of pickle. Estimated time until his airway cleared was eight to ten minutes. We began CPR in the rig and continued for about four more minutes until we arrived here."

As I filled out the PCR, the prehospital care report, for the state, I watched the ER staff do everything possible for our patient. They bagged him, used the thumper, a machine that does chest compressions, and filled his body with medications, all the while monitoring his heart. I watched the EKG screen and listened to the words exchanged among the nurses and doctors. It all added up to the same outcome. His brain had been without oxygen for too long.

When the doctor called for someone to make note of the time of death, I was not surprised. The hospital staff began its ritual of cleaning up while continuing a steady chatter on unrelated subjects.

Marge, Heather, Sam, and I completed our cleanup in the emergency room and were just walking through the ER doors when I glanced into the waiting room and saw the tiny woman, tears still streaming down her cheeks.

I usually avoid any encounter with the family when a loved one has just died. The hospital has a chaplain who comes to the ER to assist with the notification of death. But here, I suddenly felt a kinship with this woman I had met less than an hour earlier in the aisle of a supermarket.

"I know," she sobbed, looking into my eyes. "He's dead. Thanks anyway. I know you did your best."

My personal defensive wall shattered around me as my eyes met the grief-stricken eyes of this woman. Silently, I walked over and put my arms around her. I don't know how long we stood there just holding each other, and I don't know who was supporting whom. But as we stepped apart, we knew that some sort of a bond had been formed by what was now a mutual loss.

No words were ever spoken and I never saw her again. But to this day, many years later, that bond still feels as strong as ever.

On the ride back to our ambulance headquarters, tears streamed unchecked down my face, confusing the rest of the crew. Each of us builds our defenses differently, each with its distinct flaws that allow things to touch us. The scene that had so dramatically touched me had not reached my partners on the crew, and the reverse would be true on other calls.

The emotional toll on me from that call was great, but I will never regret what was exchanged between myself and the patient's loved one. I hope that I helped in her time of incredible pain, and she certainly reminded me of why I do what I do.

○ ○ ○

MY NAME IS Joan Lloyd. I'm fifty years old, tall, with curly gray hair and green eyes. Like the rest of the volunteers in the Fairfax Volunteer Ambulance Corps, FVAC,

I'm an emergency medical technician, an EMT. I am a specialist, highly trained to deal with sudden illness or injury.

We who ride with FVAC are not paramedics, so we do nothing that invades the body. We don't administer drugs or start IVs. Yet we do most of the other things that you've come to associate with paramedics. We splint, we bandage, we extricate, we do CPR, and we deliver babies. We transport patients, lights flashing and siren wailing, from the scene of sudden illness or injury, to one of several hospitals in the Fairfax area. We give comfort, a kind word, and a hand to hold. We save lives, and we watch lives slip away. And we do it without pay, but not without compensation.

Being a volunteer EMT at FVAC is a demanding profession. And it is a profession, even though we are not paid. In our state, becoming an EMT requires 110 hours of training to receive state certification and 18 more hours of defibrillation instruction to upgrade to EMT-D. Thirty or more hours are needed every three years for recertification. EMTs and paramedics are the only members of the health care profession who must recertify on a regular basis. And once the official training is completed, the real learning begins.

The Fairfax Volunteer Ambulance Corps currently boasts about 60 EMTs who volunteer at least six hours a week, carving time from their otherwise busy, full lives to help the sick and assist the injured, to comfort and cajole, to handle the silly calls and the messy ones, to laugh after the good calls and cry after the bad ones, and to provide physical and psychological first aid.

FVAC has a serious problem getting new members, particularly ones who are available daytime during the week. While we try to have crews on duty at our headquarters 24 hours a day, it gets harder and harder to find people with six hours to spend during the day. This problem, shared by most volunteer ambulance corps and rescue squads across the country, means that frequently during weekdays, our dispatchers or the police are forced to activate our paging system, which takes time. And time is our patients' worst enemy.

Ed and I both work in town and we are usually free to respond when the pagers go off. Therefore, in addition to the calls that come in during our regular shifts, we take a lot of pager calls during the day. We use two-way portable radios to communicate with others and green courtesy lights to request that drivers pull over and allow us to pass. We do not, however, violate any traffic laws in our private vehicles.

All the stories contained in this book are based on real calls. All the patients we care for, however, have a right to privacy and, although most wouldn't mind having their stories told, it would be impossible to obtain consent for this book from all of them. Therefore, in an effort to protect the privacy of all concerned, patients, relatives, and corps members, Ed and I have created the fictional town of Fairfax, a bedroom community within commuting distance of a large American city. To further disguise identities, we've fictionalized the patients' histories and often combined several calls into one. And, based on the ambulance corps with which we ride, we've created FVAC and its members.

The protocols for EMTs at FVAC and for the state certified paramedics in our stories, as well as the vehicle and traffic laws in Fairfax, are based on those of the state in which Ed and I ride. The regulations in your state may differ.

In this book, we've combined and expanded some of the hundreds of calls we've responded to over the years. We've used stories told by friends in our corps as the basis for others, telling them all as though we were there. We've also simplified the number of EMTs, often having the same EMTs respond to an unusually large number of emergencies together. Sometimes treatment in one story is not the same as in another, and often you will meet an inexperienced EMT in one story, who becomes an experienced crew chief in another. Be aware that these calls may have occurred years apart, and people have grown and protocols and equipment have changed.

This book is filled with lots of terms-of-art and abbreviations. We've tried to define each when it first occurs in the book. For translations of any of these, please refer to the section entitled "Alphabet Soup" or to the Definition of Terms at the end of the book.

Now, settle back. Learn what it's like to be an EMT and experience what we do. Ride with us and feel what it's like to respond, code 3, lights and siren, to some emergency rescue calls.

TWO

AFTER 15 YEARS of volunteer ambulance work, I still have not gotten used to the sudden transition from normal, everyday routine to life-and-death stress, then, just as suddenly, back to "normality."

It was 7:10 in the evening. Joan and I had just been seated at a table in the diner when the pager tones for an ambulance call went off and our two-way radio came alive.

"Fairfax Police to Fairfax Ambulance."

"Fairfax Ambulance on," I heard someone from headquarters answer. "Go ahead Fairfax Police."

"An ambulance is needed for a personal injury accident on the parkway, southbound, just south of Mill Street."

"10–4 Fairfax Police. Fairfax Ambulance is responding to the parkway, southbound, south of Mill Street."

Joan and I looked at each other. "Maybe we shouldn't order our dinner yet," I suggested.

"Come on, Ed," she said. "I'm starved and they don't need us. They have a full crew, and there are probably lots of people hanging around headquarters."

I was uncomfortable. Because of construction, the two directions of traffic were separated by only a low wooden divider. We had had two head-on collisions on that stretch of road within the past three months. But I remained seated, staring at the menu. Too many corps members had been "jumping" calls lately, rushing unnecessarily through town with green lights flashing. There had been complaints from local drivers, and therefore our captain had been asking people not to respond to calls unless the crew requested additional manpower.

The waitress came over to take our order.

At the next table a child in a high chair was throwing a tantrum while his parents ineffectively tried to quiet him down. "I don' wanna," the little boy shrieked, throwing his fork on the floor.

Despite the noise, Joan and I had our ears acutely tuned to our radio. It was now 7:13. "45–01 is on location," a voice I recognized as Linda Potemski's said from the radio.

The child, still shrieking, threw a spoon on the floor.

From the radio I heard, "45–01 to base." Linda sounded much too calm, like she was trying not to sound terrified.

"Ambulance base on. Go ahead 01."

"We have a head-on. There is at least one fatality and two critical injuries. We need another rig and more manpower immediately. We also need the fire department with the jaws of life."

It was now 7:14 and Joan and I were instantly on our feet. As we raced for the door, Joan shouted to the waitress, "Hold our order. We'll be back." As we ran toward my car, we could hear the honk of the fire horn from the firehouse three blocks away.

"45–22 and 45–24 are en route to the scene," I said into the radio, giving Joan's and my radio code numbers.

It was 7:17 as we approached the wreckage, green light flashing. Both ambulances, some fire apparatus, and a state trooper were already on the scene with more cars arriving each moment. We ran over to Pam Kovacs, our first lieutenant, who was standing next to one of the ambulances, microphone in hand. "What do you need?" we asked.

"I'm tied up communicating with the helicopter," she said. "It'll be here in about four minutes. I've cancelled the second rig since there's only one patient alive, but I could use your help."

"What about the jaws?" I asked. "Does anyone still need forceful extrication?"

"We'll still need the jaws to cut the two dead from their cars, Ed, but that can wait. Joan, would you walk up the parkway and find the troopers. When the helicopter is about one minute out I want you to be sure that the traffic is stopped so the chopper can land. We can keep in touch by portable."

"Will do," Joan said as she ran down the parkway and out of sight. Pam turned to me and continued, "Ed, see if you can help Linda and Pete with the patient." I was excited by the prospect of dealing with the helicopter. We had gotten emergency helicopter service only two months earlier and it would be my first experience using it.

As I ran past the two destroyed cars, I saw two bodies pinned in the wreckage, one in the driver's seat of each vehicle. Looking at the twisted metal, I was not surprised that two people were dead. I was amazed that anyone had survived such an impact. Neither car had a front end left and the passenger compartment in each car was compressed to half its original size. The passenger-side door of one car stood open, and I saw a bulky fireman replace a large pry-bar in our rig. I guessed that he and the crew had used it to force the door.

I went over to the single survivor, now lying on a longboard on the ground. Because of the hundreds of extrication calls I have been on in my 15 years with the corps, I knew that the ambulance crew had swiftly placed a cervical collar around the female patient's neck and rapidly moved her onto a backboard. They had done a full physical assessment of the seriously injured woman and had administered oxygen. I could see Linda supporting the woman's head around the bandage that covered a scalp wound.

Pete Williamson, the crew chief, was listening to the woman's lung sounds while Steve Nesbitt cut away her clothing. From the corner of my eye I could see that Phil Ortiz was bringing the MAST from one of the ambulances. Military antishock trousers, or MAST, would fit over the lower half of the woman's body and, when inflated, assist her circulation and keep her vital signs steady.

Pete looked up at me. "Ed, I want you to be committed to her airway," he said. "Don't do anything else."

"You got it, Pete," I answered.

Pete, a professional paramedic, is one of our most experienced volunteers, great to work with in any crisis. It was a shame, I often thought, that while riding with us, he was, by law, limited to EMT procedures. I knew that at this moment he wanted to start an IV line but couldn't.

I knelt next to the woman's head. Her face was covered with blood, and bits of bone or teeth jutted from her upper lip. Her age could have been anywhere from eighteen to sixty. It was impossible to tell.

"Take a deep breath," Pete told the woman as he listened to her lung sounds through his stethoscope.

To my surprise, the woman's eyes opened. She was not only conscious, but she appeared alert as well. "Can't," she cried. "Can't breathe."

"I think her trachea was partly crushed by the top of the steering wheel," Pete mouthed to me. Then to Steve, he said, "Let's get the MAST on her."

"While they do that," I said to the woman, "I'm going to help you breathe."

As Pete and the others pulled the MAST trousers on over the woman's legs, I reached for the positive-pressure oxygen mask. Removing the non-rebreather oxygen mask from her face, I began to explain the situation to her.

"We have a helicopter on the way right now," I said quietly, "and we'll have you in the hospital in five or six minutes. In the meantime, I'm going to help you breathe, but I'll need your cooperation. Every time I count to three, I am going to put this mask over your face and give you oxygen. I want you to try to inhale every time I reach three."

She tried to speak, but I stopped her. "Don't talk, just concentrate on breathing."

I counted slowly to three, placed the mask over her face and pressed the button on the positive-pressure valve, forcing air into her lungs. I could see her chest rise. "One-two-three, one-two-three." We were working together now, in a regular rhythm.

I repeated the process again and again, helping her get the oxygen that she desperately needed for survival. "One-two-three."

The antishock trousers were now in place, and Phil was using the foot pump to inflate them. "I'm not waiting for the helicopter," Pete said, his calm voice belying his obvious impatience. "When the MAST is inflated, strap her onto the stretcher and load her into the ambulance. If the damn chopper isn't here by the time we're ready, we're going to roll."

As the moments passed, the woman was becoming agitated and was no longer cooperating with me as I attempted to assist her breathing. "I feel like I'm choking when you put the mask over my face," she said, pushing my hand away with her one free arm.

"It's helping you breathe," I responded. "You need the oxygen."

"No, please stop. I can't stand the feeling," she pleaded.

Pete had stretched Velcro straps across the woman's body to secure it to the board, and Linda had taped down the woman's head, with headblocks on either side to keep her head from moving. We were ready to move the stretcher, and while in motion it would have been difficult to continue to use the positive-pressure mask anyway. "Okay," I said to her. "I'll put the other mask back on you for the moment."

I placed the non-rebreather mask back on her face and started to push the stretcher toward the rig. Suddenly, I became aware of a pulsating sound from above. Looking up, I saw the steel bird circle once, then descend toward us, its lifesaving skilike talons reaching for the pavement of the parkway.

"It's going to get windy!" Steve yelled. We huddled over our patient to protect her from the blast of wind from the rotors and the debris kicked up by the prop wash.

Suddenly the helicopter was down and two flight nurses were with us, starting an IV line and instructing us as to how to load the patient into the chopper.

It was 7:24 when the helicopter lifted off the parkway on its four-minute flight to St. Luke's Trauma Center. There was nothing more either Joan or I could do.

At 7:30 Joan and I arrived back at the restaurant. Our table was still empty. The child at the next table was still throwing his tantrum. "Gimme that," he screamed at his cowed parents, grabbing a handful of ice cream from his mother's plate.

At 7:32 the waitress brought us our chicken and tacos and we began to eat our dinner.

○ ○ ○

MY NAME IS Ed Herman and I'm fifty-five years old. I've been a member of the Fairfax Volunteer Ambulance Corps for 15 years and I enjoy it more today than I did when I started.

Why become an EMT?

In my early teens, when I was just beginning to really take an interest in girls, I went to a school picnic. Around lunchtime a very pretty girl in my class named Rochelle, but who everyone called "Rocky," was wading in a stream near the picnic area. Suddenly she began to scream. She had stepped on a piece of glass and had cut her foot badly. One of the older boys rushed into the stream, picked her up, and carried her to the nearby first-aid station.

I wished that I had been that boy.

Over the next few weeks, I read every first-aid book I could find and fantasized about myself rushing in to rescue some injured person (preferably a pretty girl). I would be the most important person around because I would be the only one who knew what to do. Sometimes the treatment would be painful, but I would always be able to comfort whomever I was rescuing (again, preferably a pretty girl).

These fantasies somehow mingled with earlier childhood fantasies of being the Lone Ranger—arriving on the scene on a white horse, "just in the nick of time" so to speak (preferably to rescue a pretty girl). Part of the Lone Ranger fantasy was that, like him, I could act outside the law, with almost godlike powers.

Now, when the claxon at ambulance headquarters sounds, I jump into my white ambulance. When I drive the rig, I am immune from most traffic laws. I sometimes arrive at the scene in the "nick of time," although more often there is no great emergency involved. And sometimes I arrive too late.

When I am crew chief or the first EMT on the scene of a serious illness or injury, I am, at that moment, the most important person in the world. Everyone, including the police, await and abide by my decisions. At that place and time, no king has greater power or responsibility. And almost always I am able, to a greater or lesser degree, to provide comfort to sick, injured, or frightened people (although they are rarely young attractive females).

How many people can come so close to attaining their childhood fantasies?

THE CORPS MEMBERS, POLICE OFFICERS, AND OTHER CHARACTERS IN THIS BOOK

YOU'VE ALREADY MET some of the members of the Fairfax Volunteer Ambulance Corps, and you'll meet many more. You'll also meet firefighters and police officers who live and work in Fairfax and in other nearby towns.

To help you remember the characters in this book, below is a listing of the members of FVAC, the Fairfax Police Department, Prescott Rescue Squad, and the Prescott Police Department. I've also included some of the doctors and nurses we work with and a few other characters you'll encounter. All of these people are fictional composites of the people with whom we ride.

Fairfax Volunteer Ambulance Corps

Radio Call GKL-642
County prefix 45

Emergency Medical Technicians

Nick Abrams—age thirty-four—works split shifts at the local Mobil station.

Stephanie DiMartino—age twenty-one—works in the local K Mart.

Bob Fiorella—age thirty-five—sells insurance and is able to respond to day calls when he's in the area.

Heather Franks—age twenty-four—works in the lunchroom of George Washington Elementary School and goes to college part-time.

Tom Franks—age twenty-five—Heather's husband and a second-grade teacher at John Adams Elementary school in Fairfax.

Dave Hancock—age thirty-one—FVAC's Maintenance officer—auto mechanic at a local auto-body shop.

Ed Herman—age fifty-five—publisher and biotechnology specialist who works from his home. Radio call number is 45–22.

Pam Kovacs—first lieutenant—age thirty-eight—works part-time for a florist. Radio call number 45–12.

Joan Lloyd—age fifty—writer who works at home and responds to day calls. Radio call number 45–24.

Judy Lloyd—age twenty-four—rode with FVAC for four years before moving to the southwest.

Jack McCaffrey—age forty-five—professor at Fairfax Community College.

Sam Middleton—age twenty-seven—city firefighter—rides variable shifts as they fit into his schedule.

Steve Nesbitt—age fifty-one—drives a school bus for the Fairfax school system.

Phil Ortiz—age eighteen—became a first responder in the youth corps then, when he became eighteen, he advanced to the senior squad and became an EMT.

Linda Potemski—age thirty-nine—emergency room nurse at Fairfax Hospital and a longtime member of FVAC.

Fred Stevens—age forty-two—electrician with a local construction firm.

Marge Talbot—age thirty-four—CPA with a large accounting firm. Frequently works via computer modem and thus can occasionally respond to day calls.

Jill Tremonte—age twenty—dental assistant with the Fairfax Dental Group.

Pete Williamson—age twenty-five—professional paramedic with an EMS service in the city.

Probationary members

Tim Babbett—age twenty-three—works for a local contractor—an EMT but hasn't yet become a full member of the corps.

Davida Herman—age nineteen—member of the youth group who graduated to the senior corps as a probationary member on her eighteenth birthday.

Dispatcher

Greg Horvath—age sixty-eight—retired plumber.

Fairfax Police Department

Radio Call ID GBY-639

Officers

Merve Berkowitz car 317
Chuck Harding car 305
Will McAndrews car 312
Stan Poritsky car 308
Detective Irv Greenberg

Dispatcher

Mark Thomas

Prescott Volunteer Rescue Squad

County prefix 21

Members

Paramedic Amy Chen
Paramedic Hugh Washington
EMT Sally Walsh

Prescott Police Department

Radio Call ID GRQ-325

Officers

Stan Garth car 715
Mike Gold car 706
Roy Zimmerman car 703

At Fairfax General Hospital ER

Dr. Frank Margolis—emergency medicine specialist.
Kurt Bankcroft RN—emergency room nurse.
Rosemary Harper RN—emergency room head nurse.

At Oakside Psychiatric Center

Dr. Susan Cardone—psychiatrist and crisis specialist.

At St. Luke's Trauma Center

Dr. Robert Englander—trauma specialist.

THREE

IT WAS MID-AFTERNOON, in the midst of a violent summer thunderstorm, when the call came in on my scanner.

"Fairfax Police to Fairfax Ambulance. The ambulance is needed for a serious personal injury auto accident on Route 10 at the bad curve."

"10–4, Fairfax Police." I recognized the voice of Greg Horvath, a retired plumber who dispatched for us on Tuesday afternoons. "45–01 is responding with an EMT and a driver. I'll be paging out for at least one more member."

"10–4. Be advised that we also have an officer en route."

Sitting at my desk at home, I quickly considered several factors. First, I hate thunderstorms. Since childhood I have had an unreasonable fear of lightning, and the flashes were coming frequently now. Second, it was pouring—big, fat drops soaking everyone and everything foolish enough to be out in it. In addition, I was in the middle of writing a magazine article and I hate to be interrupted.

Before the dispatcher had a chance to press the pager key, however, I had picked up the phone and pressed the auto-dialer button for corps headquarters. As I heard the phone ring, I admitted to myself that I'm addicted.

"Fairfax Ambulance," Greg answered from headquarters.

"This is Joan Lloyd. Tell 01 that I'll meet them at the scene."

"10–4, Joan. I've heard several more reports on the CB. I'm going to page for a standby crew."

"Good idea, Greg. Just in case."

I drove toward the bad curve on route 10, doing only 30 miles per hour on the rain-slick pavement. I started to plug in the green light I have on the roof of my car but stopped myself. I didn't want any cars making sudden moves and possibly causing another accident.

As I drove, I could hear Greg tone out for additional members to respond to the scene and a standby crew for the second rig. If the accident was truly serious, we were going to need manpower, a rare commodity on a weekday afternoon.

I saw the flares before I saw the cars. A tall, slender man in heavy work boots was setting up a flare pattern, warning oncoming traffic of the wreck. I saw no familiar cars. Neither other corps members nor police were on the scene yet.

I pulled my car off the roadway and keyed the mike on my portable radio. "45–24 is on location." As I got out of my car I realized that the rain had become only a light drizzle. I had been so focused on the accident that I had no idea when the lightning had stopped.

"10–4, 24," Greg said. "Let me know if you'll need a second rig."

Two cars, a black Honda Prelude and a dark blue station wagon, were about 20 feet apart. Both had severe front-end damage. There were several people standing around with that helpless look that has become so familiar to me over the years. People at an accident scene are always eager to help; they just don't know what to do.

"How many injured?" I called. I needed to know as quickly as possible how many ambulances we might need.

"There's a man in that car," one man said, pointing to the Honda. "His face is bleeding and he says that his neck and head hurt."

I heard only the phrase "he says." The man in the Honda was obviously conscious and alert so his injuries were probably not immediately life threatening. "Someone try to keep him from moving around. I want to see what we have in the other car." Two young women trotted toward the Honda, happy that they now had something constructive to do.

"There's a woman and two children in the station wagon," a man said. As I sprinted toward the open driver's side window, I heard a child in the passenger front seat crying.

"Hi," I said to the woman behind the wheel. "My name's Joan and I'm with the ambulance corps. I need you to hold very still and be patient for a few moments longer. Where do you hurt?"

"It's my chest," she said. "And my daughter says she can't breathe."

"What happened?" I asked, my hands quickly assessing her head, neck, and ribs.

"I tried to turn, but the car wouldn't." She was responding to my questions, her color was good, and my hands found nothing severe, so I decided that her injuries could wait for a few minutes.

"Seat belts?" I asked as I opened her door slightly, then relatched it. I didn't want to open it fully yet because that would move the driver, but I now knew it would open when we needed it. For the moment, it was better to keep her still until I had more help.

"Oh, yes, we were all belted. How are my kids?"

"I'll check out your children right now. Just don't move." I saw one little girl in the front passenger seat and another lying on the seat in the back, both looking at me with huge, tear-filled eyes.

Four patients. We'd need at least two rigs. As I keyed my mike, I became aware of a welcome siren as the approaching first ambulance rolled to a stop, followed immediately by a police car. "45–24 to base."

"Base on."

"We have four injuries. Roll that second rig as soon as you have a driver. Have any additional personnel respond to the scene." I clipped the radio back on to my front jeans pocket.

"10–4, Joan. 45–02 will be responding in about thirty seconds."

As two crew members climbed out of the duty rig, I pointed. "I haven't assessed the man in that car. A bystander said that he's conscious, complaining of head and neck pain. The woman who was driving this car and her two little girls are conscious as well."

Heather Franks ran to care for the man, while Nick Abrams, the driver, began to get the equipment we'd need from the rig. Stan Portisky, a Fairfax policeman I had worked with often, was quickly returning order to the scene and directing traffic around the accident.

I ran around to the passenger side of the car and directed my attention to the whimpering girl in the front seat. The front window was open, but as I pulled at the door handle, I realized that her door was jammed shut.

I immediately realized that, unless we could force this door, the mother would have to be extricated before the girl. I briefly considered calling for the fire department and their jaws of life, but it would take time for them to assemble a crew and it would be terrifying for the children. I decided that because none of the patients appeared to be critical, their condition gave us enough time to remove the mother, then her daughter, through the driver's side door. The second girl could be removed from the back quickly, because both back doors appeared to be undamaged.

I waved at Nick, now pulling equipment from the rig, and called, "Bring an oxygen bottle for this nice woman and one for the girl in the front seat."

"Sure," Nick yelled. "Coming up."

"Hi, sweetheart. What's your name?" I asked the little girl who was softly weeping in the front seat. I wanted to hear her speak so I could determine if she had any respiratory problems.

"Her name is Patricia," came a small voice from the backseat. The older girl, lying across the backseat behind her mother, had a huge bluish egg rising above her left eye. I pulled at the back door and, as I had suspected, it opened easily. With as little movement to the car as possible, I slipped into the backseat and quickly reached one arm around each side of the front seat and ran my hands over the whimpering younger girl.

"Okay, Patricia, try not to cry." *I don't feel anything serious yet,* I thought, *and, if you can cry, you're not having too much trouble breathing.* I returned to the girl in the backseat. "And what's your name?"

"I'm Linda and my mother is Nancy."

"Where do you hurt?"

"My face, my stomach, and my legs," she said, making a supreme effort not to cry as her sister was doing. "And I'm getting a bad headache."

"Well, you and your family are being very brave and that's very important right now. We're here to take the best care of you, but you have to hang in there for a few minutes. Just hold very still and don't move."

"Okay," Linda nodded.

"I don't even want you to nod your head," I said. I caught the eye of a middle-aged man in a three-piece suit who was standing next to the car. The rain had finally stopped, but the man was soaked to the skin. "Sir, can you help me and open the back door on the other side?"

"I guess." He ran around to the driver's side.

When I saw him reach for the door handle, I added, "We don't want to jiggle the car any more than we have to, so I need you to do things very gently." Carefully he opened the door.

"That's great." I motioned toward Linda, stretched out across the backseat. "Now, can you hold this lovely young lady's head? We need to remind her not to move."

The man looked a bit bewildered, but he did as I had asked, placing one palm against each side of Linda's face.

Nancy kept looking around to assure herself that her children were all right. "Ma'am," I said, "you have to hold as still as you can. I'll be in charge of your girls."

My arms contorted around the front seat, I pressed my palm against Patricia's forehead. The most important thing that can be done for victims of violent trauma is to prevent any additional injury until there are enough hands to do a full immobilization. "Patricia," I said to her. "That's a big name for a little girl. What do your friends call you? Patty or Patsy?"

"Patricia," she said firmly. She had obviously been asked that question many times.

"Okay. Patricia it is."

In addition to placing a collar bag, a KED tape and straps within easy reach, Nick had attached a non-rebreather face mask to a portable oxygen cylinder. He set the cylinder's flow at 12 liters per minute and placed the mask on the driver's face. Then he walked around to the passenger side, reached through the window, and placed a second tank, with a pediatric mask attached, on the front seat near the door.

"It's here whenever you need this," he said to me. "What now?"

"Stay right there for a minute," I answered. "Patricia," I said to the girl, still whimpering in the front seat, "can you talk to me?" I squeezed her shoulder gently, lending her my support.

"I guess so," the tiny voice said.

"That's great. You're doin' good." I sighed gratefully as I saw the flashing green lights of other members' cars arriving at the scene. Now I could use Nick and free up my hands. "Nick, can you hold Patricia's head for me and help her with some oxygen?"

"Sure." Nick reached in through the window and held the little girl's forehead with one hand and held the oxygen mask near her face with the other. Sometimes children become frightened when we fasten a mask over their face, so we try to hold the mask rather than tighten the elastic band around their head.

I unwound my arms from the front seat and twisted my head to release the tension in my neck and shoulders. "Girls," I said, "just stay still now and we'll help you very soon." I softly stroked Linda's cheek and checked her carotid pulse. Pulse good and strong, skin warm and dry. All good so far. "Darling, I'm going to touch your body. I need you to tell me if anything I do hurts. Okay?"

Quickly, I ran my hands over her neck, chest, arms, and legs and was glad when she didn't complain of any pain. When, I palpated her abdomen gently, she winced. "Ow, that hurts."

"I'm sorry if I hurt you, Linda. I won't touch you there again." Pain and tenderness in the two lower abdominal quadrants. Probably seat belt trauma with possible internal injury. Then I pressed gently on her scalp, cheekbones, and jaw, carefully avoiding the huge, multicolored lump over her right eye. No point tenderness, a good sign.

"Now," I said as I finished my brief survey, "we have a few minutes to talk. How old are you, Linda?"

"I'm nine," she said. "And my sister's . . ."

"Let's see if she can tell me how old she is." Other crew members began to crawl around us, as they fully immobilized the mother so she could be extricated from the wreckage.

"I'm five," Patricia said through her tears and around the oxygen mask Nick still held.

"Well, ladies, you're both being very grown up. This is pretty scary, but you're doing just fine. Are either of you married?"

I love asking little children off-the-wall questions like that. They inevitably think that I've lost my mind. Then sometimes they giggle or get indignant, but whatever their reaction, they begin to relax.

"No," both girls said, simultaneously. Then Linda said, "We're too little to be married. Are you married?"

As the three of us talked, I reached around the front seat and did a more thorough survey of Patricia's small body while Nick continued to secure her head. She winced as I touched her chest and abdomen but the rest of her body seemed uninjured. "Does your chest hurt a lot?" I asked.

"Yes," she said, her lower lip quivering. "And my tummy, too."

Hoping that she would believe, I said, "Well, that oxygen should help the pain."

"How are my girls?" Nancy asked as the crew prepared her for transfer to a long spine board. Her head was already restrained in the KED, so she could see only straight ahead. "Are they really all right?"

"They're doing fine," I answered. "They both have injuries from the seat belts, and Linda has a very colorful egg on her forehead, but otherwise they're doin' good. What do you say, girls?"

"We're okay, mom," Linda said. "It hurts, but we're okay."

"Patricia," I said, "I think mommy would like to hear you say you're all right."

"I'm okay, Mommy. I'm being brave."

"You sure are," I said.

Nick was hunched over, still leaning in through the window in a very contorted position. I reached around and held Patricia's head, freeing one of Nick's arms. Because Patricia seemed to be moving her arms and legs without difficulty and because I know it always makes people feel better if they have some control over what's going on around them, I suggested, "Patricia. That oxygen should be helping and I think you're big enough to hold it all by yourself. What do you think?"

"Okay. I could hold it, I think." Nick handed the mask to her, and she proudly held it against her face. "I do feel better," Patricia said. Thank heavens for the power of suggestion. Frequently, that and psychological first aid are all we have.

We continued talking as calmly as we could, while turmoil whirled around us. Through what was left of the front windshield, I could see Heather and three members of the crew of the second rig doing a full immobilization of the man in the Honda.

As Nancy was removed from the car, I said to the girls, "They are going to put your mom into the ambulance, then we're going to get you out. It will take a bit more time, but we can be patient, can't we?"

"I guess," they said.

"You know, I think we have a couple of bears in the ambulance who might like some new people to love them. One for each of you. While we wait, we have to think of names for them. That's a very important job, naming bears." While the crews worked, the three of us deliberated, selecting and discarding bear names.

"What about Terwilliger," I suggested. "When I was little, I used to have a stuffed turtle named Terwilliger."

"That's a silly name," Patricia said softly from the front seat.

"My turtle liked it. Maybe the bear will think it's a great name," I said. "As a matter of fact, maybe we should let him help choose his own name."

"Maybe," she said. "But bears can't think so good."

It took still more time to get collars on both children. We slid Linda across the backseat, directly onto a long backboard, then put Patricia on a shorter board and took her out through the driver's side door. When everyone was loaded, I ended up in one ambulance with the man from the Honda, Heather, who had been caring for him, Nick, and Patricia. Linda and her mother were in the other ambulance with the crew of the second rig.

I searched the rig for a bear for Patricia, and finally found one in the pediatric bag. He was about six inches tall, brown, and fluffy, with a plaid bow tie. I showed the small soft animal to the brave little girl and said, "I just asked him and this bear thinks Terwilliger is a great name. Terwilliger, meet Patricia." I tucked him into the crook of Patricia's arm. "You can keep him forever, you know. I think he'll like living with a girl as brave as you are."

"Thanks, Joan." She wrapped her arm around the bear and seemed to be resting easily. "Will my sister get a bear, too, just like this?"

"Not all our stuffies are the same. When you get to the hospital, you'll have to see what kind Linda got and what she named him."

Patricia gave me a weak smile. "Terwilliger's the best bear with the best name."

During the ride to the hospital, I worried about Patricia. I had detected increasing abdominal rigidity, but at least she was breathing comfortably. Also I was afraid that she would become anxious, being separated from her mother, but, hugging her bear, she quickly fell asleep. I rechecked her pulse and respirations several times and was pleased that her vitals remained stable.

When we arrived at the hospital, it was controlled bedlam. Because of the rainstorm, there had been several other accidents and the staff was stretched thin. Despite that, they were wonderful with the children, and I felt I was leaving them in good hands. After I finished my paperwork, I slipped into Patricia's cubicle and kissed her on the forehead. "Goodbye," I said. "Give Terwilliger an extra hug for me."

"I will," she said.

I found Linda in a room down the hall. She showed me the light-blue stuffed whale she had been given by her ambulance crew. "May I keep him?"

"You sure can. And wait till you see your sister's bear. His name is Terwilliger."

"Thanks, Joan. Thanks for taking care of us."

I located Nancy, still strapped to the long spine board, on a gurney in the hall. "Your girls are in good shape," I told her, "and they're being well taken care of so you can relax."

"Are they really okay?"

"They don't seem to have anything too serious, but I don't have X-ray eyes. I've already made sure that Dr. Margolis knows that you're their mother, and he'll keep you informed."

"Thanks so much. I don't know how we would have gotten through this without you." She smiled at me and that made everything I do with the ambulance worthwhile.

The following day, I returned to the hospital to pick up the assortment of equipment we had left there. I discovered that, while the man from the Honda had been treated and released, Linda, Patricia, and their mother had all been admitted. I took a few minutes and went up to visit Nancy.

As I introduced myself, she said, "I remember you. You were at the accident."

"I certainly was, but sometimes people don't remember those things very well. How are you?"

"I hurt all over," she said, "but I'm going to be fine. They say I may have bruised my heart, and I have lots of small cuts and scrapes. Patricia has a bruised liver. They were very happy that she didn't rupture her spleen. Linda fractured one of the bones in her face and she had some trauma to her lower abdomen."

"Thank God you were wearing seat belts," I said.

"You really think so? The doctor said some of our injuries are seat belt related. Do you really think we're better off?"

"Think about it," I said. "If the impact was hard enough for the seat belts to do that kind of damage, imagine what would have happened if you and the children hadn't been buckled. Patricia would have been thrown out through the front window, probably followed by Linda. You would have crushed your chest on the steering wheel and quite possibly put your face through the front windshield."

"I guess that's right," she said in a small voice.

"Don't ever let your children ride without their belts. Please, promise me."

She promised. I hope she doesn't decide some time in the future that she and the girls would have been better off without those lifesaving seat belts. Everyone seems to know an anecdote about someone who was better off without a seat belt, and they use that story as an excuse not to buckle. No one seems to have anecdotes about the thousands of people whose lives have been saved by seat belts.

○ ○ ○

EVERY YEAR, THE county gives awards to ambulance and rescue crews, police and fire personnel who have done something extraordinary. Many of the awards are given for saves, of which there are several dozen each year. The number of people brought back to life after cardiac arrest is amazingly small, though, considering the number of calls logged in the county each year.

At the awards ceremony, everyone involved, no matter how nonchalant he wants to appear, is honored and thrilled to have been a part of saving a life. Dave Hancock and Jill Tremonte and I, and Fairfax police officer Will McAndrews, will receive awards this year.

Early one Tuesday afternoon, my crew and I were called to the home of a "man down." When we arrived, we were met at the door by a hysterical woman, yelling, "Do something, please!"

"Where?"

"In there." She motioned toward the bedroom at the end of the hall. "I can't wake my husband, Carlos, up."

As my crew and I ran into the bedroom, Officer Will McAndrews was attempting to get the overweight man from the bed onto the floor. We all put our equipment down and, with Will at the head, Dave and me at the man's waist and Jill at the feet, dragged the man onto the gold bedroom rug. I assembled the bag mask and hooked up the oxygen.

Dave checked the man's breathing and pulse, shook his head and said, "Will, do compressions and I'll ventilate."

Because I was crew chief I let Dave and Will begin CPR while I set up the defibrillator, a device that can "jump start" a stopped heart. I had to stay back and remain aware of the entire scene.

Dave slipped an airway into the man's mouth, took the bag-valve-mask, pressed the attached mask to the man's face, and began to squeeze the bag to ventilate, while Will began to compress the man's chest. "One, two, three, four, five." Dave squeezed the bag, forcing life-preserving oxygen into the man's lungs.

"Take my radio," I said to Jill, "and ask the police to get us some more help. At least one more person, two if possible."

While I pulled the electrodes from the defibrillator case and put the recording tape and module into the machine, I could hear Jill saying, "45–01 to Fairfax police. Tone out for two additional members to respond to this scene for a code 99." Code 99. CPR in progress.

"Jill," I said as she finished, "get the stretcher and a long spine board. He's so heavy, we'll need to use the board to lift him onto the stretcher."

I attached the large defibrillator pads, one to his upper right chest, the other under his left ribs, and spoke into the machine to record the information. "This is EMT Joan Lloyd. CPR is in progress on a . . ." I turned to his wife. "How old is your husband?"

"He's seventy-three, and he's had two previous heart attacks and three minor strokes."

As I turned back to the machine and recorded the relevant information, I thought, *This isn't going to work. With that history, he's a bad candidate for a save.*

"Everyone stop CPR," I said as I pushed the "Press to Analyze" button and looked at the screen. "He's in course V-fib." Ventricular fibrillation is a disorganized heart motion that is incapable of circulating enough blood to keep a body alive. The rising whine of the machine indicated that it was charging, preparing to allow me to deliver a shock that might convert his rhythm to "normal sinus," the regular rhythm of a working heart.

"Stand clear," I yelled as the robotlike voice of the machine intoned, "Press to Shock, Press to Shock." Will and Dave moved back, away from any contact with the patient. I quickly searched for my patient's carotid pulse and found none. I pressed the button and watched as the man's body reacted violently to the 200 watt-seconds of current passing through his body. I studied the screen and pressed the analyze button again. "Still V-fib," I said and repeated the process, delivering a second shock.

The rhythm on the screen now appeared to be a sinus rhythm, but it was only about ten beats per minute, too slow to be doing any good. I felt no pulse in the man's neck. I suspected EMD, electromechanical dissociation. His heart was giving off electrical signals that weren't triggering any heart-muscle movement, any actual beats. There was little more we, as EMTs, could do.

"Continue CPR and let's transport."

We continued CPR as we loaded the man into the rig. Because no one else had been available, we pressed Will McAndrews into service as driver, and rushed, code 3, to the hospital.

At the hospital we turned the patient over to the Emergency Room staff, who were ready to "work the code" and try to restore life to our clinically dead patient.

"Talk to me," the ER doctor said as we wheeled the man in.

"We shocked twice and converted to a pulseless sinus rhythm, rate about ten. I suspect EMD. He has a history of two previous heart attacks and three strokes. Approximate downtime before CPR three minutes." I glanced at my watch. "Total time since he went down, about twenty-three minutes."

Once we finished cleaning up, we called the police to let them know that we would respond from the hospital if any other calls came in. Then we stood out of the way. There didn't seem to be any hope, but we couldn't resist staying to see what happened. As I watched, the ER staff gave the patient medications and monitored his EKG. After about half an hour, I was amazed to see that his EKG looked almost normal.

"That looks like a good rhythm," I mumbled.

"It is," one of the nurses told me. "So far so good. He's breathing on his own and his blood pressure is ninety over sixty-five."

"You mean he's going to make it?"

"Very possibly. You didn't have EMD, Joan," Dr. Margolis explained as he worked. "You had a slow but viable rhythm that we could work with. Between his weak beats and your crew's good CPR, you got him here with enough oxygen in his system to maintain him. We'll monitor for a while here, and if he remains stable we'll send him up to CCU."

"Holy shit," I muttered. "Holy shit."

Totally elated, I shared the good news with my crew, wrote up the paperwork, and returned to headquarters. We were all flying. A save is the most wonderful feeling in the world.

On the TV show *Rescue 911*, after a successful rescue, the crew and the patient often become good friends and live happily ever after. I wish that had been true in this case. I stayed in touch with the hospital and found out that the man died eight days later of another massive heart attack. Although I wish the outcome had been otherwise, I found that his death didn't diminish my elation at having saved him.

Almost three months later, Ed and I were having dinner in the Fairfax Diner when a woman came over to our table and sat down. Although she looked familiar, I didn't recognize her at first.

"I'm sure you don't remember me, but you saved my husband, Carlos Perez."

"Mrs. Perez," I said. "I'm so glad to see you." I introduced her to Ed, then said, "I was sorry to hear about your husband."

"You and your crew gave us all an extra week. I called our son and daughter-in-law and they flew home. They live in the southwest, and I'm moving down there in a month or so. Anyway, we all gathered at the hospital and had a last chance to be together as a family. A lot of good things came out of that week, and I'll be forever grateful for it."

I swallowed the lump in my throat as the woman rose. "Thank you again for everything," she said. "And thank your crew."

"I will." I stood and we hugged. I don't expect to see her again.

On TV the rescuer always says, modestly, that he isn't a hero. I guess that's true, in a way. I was in the right place at the right time, doing the job I was trained to do. But I was there when I was needed, and my training and the ability to put it into action helped save a person's life. That's a wonderful feeling and, hero or not, I will proudly wear the red and white pin that I will receive from the county as a symbol of my save.

○ ○ ○

IT BEGAN WHEN Tom and Laura Conklin left their three-year-old son in the care of Tom's mother while they went away for a well-deserved weekend vacation. Mrs. Conklin had often baby-sat for Jeremy and spent the weekend playing with the active youngster. On Sunday afternoon, when Jeremy and his grandmother returned from a trip to the store, Mrs. Conklin parked the car at the top of the sloping driveway.

"Lemme drive, Gramma. Lemme drive."

"Okay, darling. Let's take the groceries into the house, then you can drive." Together Jeremy and Mrs. Conklin carried groceries into the kitchen and put them away. "I wanna drive now. You promised Gramma."

They walked out to the car, and Mrs. Conklin put Jeremy behind the wheel. "Okay," Jeremy said. "We're racing down the road." Mrs. Conklin stood beside the open car door while her grandson grabbed the steering wheel and pretended to drive.

The police never found out whether the hand brake failed or had never been set, but when Jeremy suddenly knocked the gearshift into neutral, the car started to roll backward. Screaming, Mrs. Conklin quickly snatched the boy from the driver's seat and attempted to pull him to safety. But her arm was hit by the open driver's side door, and she dropped Jeremy beneath the front wheels. The blow to his head was a glancing one, but when she picked him up from the driveway, despite the lack of blood, she knew that his injury was serious.

"Oh, God," she moaned. "Oh, God."

The car had stopped rolling, and Mrs. Conklin grabbed the child and placed him across the front passenger's seat. For reasons we never quite understood, she drove to the Texaco station at the main intersection in town. There, one of the employees phoned the police, and they, in turn, called for the ambulance.

"Fairfax Police to Fairfax Ambulance. An ambulance is needed at the Texaco station at the intersection of Routes 10 and 51 for a child who has been struck by a car."

I heard the tones from my apartment about a quarter of a mile from the center of town. Because there is seldom a crew on a Sunday afternoon and I knew lots of help might be needed, I yelled to my daughter, Judy, who at that time also rode with the corps. "You coming?"

"Right behind you, Mom."

I called the police to let them know that two EMTs were responding, and we both jumped into my car. It took only 30 seconds to cover the short distance to the center of town. As soon as I pulled into the Texaco station, I saw a crowd gathered around a small figure lying on the ground.

Judy pointed toward an older woman sitting in the front seat of a car, weeping. "I'll take care of her," Judy yelled. "You see to the boy."

As Judy ran over to the older woman to ascertain whether she was injured, I elbowed my way through the crush of people gathered around the little boy. I will never forget the sight. He was lying on the ground, unresponsive, dressed in a red and white polo shirt, red shorts and white socks with red stripes. To this day, when I see a little boy dressed that way I swallow hard and flash back to that afternoon.

"What happened?" I yelled.

"Don't know. That woman was carrying him when I drove in," a man in the crowd said. "She looked like she was going to faint, so I took him from her and laid him down here."

I did a quick examination and found that the boy had stopped breathing and had no pulse. I began CPR immediately. I have no recollection of how long it was before the rig arrived, but it seemed like forever. I had no idea what had happened or whether there were others injured. I just focused on doing CPR.

When the rig arrived, I remember that Phil Ortiz, one of our younger members, and I lifted the boy onto a short wooden spine board and we continued CPR, in silence, all the way to the hospital. I didn't even know who was driving. I just watched Phil compress the boy's little chest while I used a pediatric BVM to blow oxygen-enriched air into his lungs. We sped to the hospital, siren screaming, each knowing privately that there was no hope. Recovery from cardiac arrest due to trauma is almost impossible, especially when the victim is a child.

I found out later that Judy accompanied the boy's grandmother to the hospital in a second ambulance. As my daughter explained later the ambulance was unnecessary for physical reasons. Psychologically, though, it seemed to help the older woman.

When we got to Fairfax General, the closest hospital, we transferred care of our patient to the ER staff, but it was no use. We stood and watched until the doctor pronounced the little boy dead 45 minutes later.

Today there is a team of professional counselors who can be called upon to help crew members deal with the emotional stress of a difficult call. The process, called critical incident stress debriefing, didn't exist at that time, so we had to cope on our own. My daughter's boyfriend met her at headquarters, and I called Ed, who picked me up at the hospital.

As an EMT, I have learned to deal with death. Most of the calls I go on involve people I don't know. When I don't know someone alive, *I have little emotional reaction in seeing him after death.* But with a child, things are different.

I cried over this call. I cried for the waste. I remember saying, "Little kids shouldn't die." I cried for the boy's grandmother who would have to live with this for the rest of her life. I cried for the child's parents who didn't even know yet what had happened. I cried for myself. I had felt so helpless. And the whole thing seemed so senseless. So totally senseless.

○ ○ ○

IT WAS ABOUT seven-thirty on a Wednesday evening. Ted Fredrickson and his son Scotty were driving south on the parkway that runs through Fairfax. The engine of the car had been coughing and sputtering for 20 miles, and Ted had been driving slowly with his flashers on.

"Dad," Scotty said, "why don't we find a gas station and call Mom."

"No need to bother your mother," Ted said. "We'll be home in just a few minutes, and I'm sure that the car can hold out until then."

"But, Dad," Scotty pressed, "you're doing only about thirty in a fifty-five-mile zone."

"Don't worry. We'll be fine."

The car made it to a point about halfway across the bridge over the reservoir, then conked out completely. Ted rolled to a stop in the center lane and left his flashers on so that cars could see him and pass on either side.

Ted cranked the engine several times, then unsnapped his seat belt. "Damn," he sighed, zipping his down jacket. "You stay here and I'll see if I can get this thing started."

Ted waited until the fast lane of traffic was clear, then got out, walked around to the front of the car, and raised the hood to try to repair the damage. He never saw the small van that plowed into the rear end of his car.

"You fuckin' idiot," the man who had been driving the van yelled as he ran up beside the driver's window a moment later. "What the hell do you mean stopping in the center lane? I could have been killed." But there was no one in the driver's seat.

Scotty, unhurt, gathered his wits and peered through the space between the windshield wipers and the edge of the raised hood for his father. Ted had disappeared.

"My dad!" he shrieked. "Where's my dad?"

"Fairfax Police to the ambulance. Dispatch an ambulance to the southbound parkway bridge over the reservoir for a serious PIAA," my portable radio squawked.

"10–4," the voice from headquarters said. "45–01 is responding. Tone out for one more member to meet us at the scene." I quickly called in to say that I was responding.

"10–4, Joan. 45–01 will meet you there." I recognized Pam Kovacs's voice and was glad that she would be there. She was always calm in a crisis and, since she'd been elected first lieutenant, she'd gained a lot of authority.

Although there was a foot or so of old snow covering the grassy areas beside the parkway, the roads were clear and I made good time. I arrived at the scene just after the rig. As I got out of my car, I saw that Sam Middleton was examining the driver of the van. He quickly gave the thumbs-up sign, which indicated that the man was uninjured.

In addition to being an EMT, Tom Franks, another crew member, was also a second-grade schoolteacher. "Tom," Pam said as she pointed to Scotty, "stay with the boy and keep him away from what's happening." With a fatherly arm around the boy's shoulder, Tom escorted Scotty to a warm police car.

"What's going on?" I asked, each word coming out with a little puff of frozen air.

"From what the police can find out, the kid's dad was in front of the car when it was hit. Looks like he went over the side of the bridge and down the embankment."

"Oh, shit," I said.

"Yeah," Pam said.

"You know he could be in the reservoir."

"Let's not think about that yet."

"Yeah, but if he's in the water, we'll have to call the divers," I said as we removed two powerful flashlights from the rig.

"I think they've already got them coming, but if the man's in the reservoir, there's not much chance he's still alive. Let's see if we can find him on the embankment." Pam and I joined the police and played the lights over the snow-covered landscape beside the reservoir. I wasn't sure

I wanted to see what was there. The ground, at least 50 feet below us, was covered with snow; rocks and trees made dark shadows so we didn't know exactly what we were seeing.

Soon we were joined by the fire department with heavy-duty floodlights. I saw two engines arriving via the fire road around the reservoir at the foot of the embankment. They parked below us and played search lights on the snow and the road.

After about ten minutes someone on the road below called, "Here! We found something." We could see their lights focusing on a spot about 60 feet below us, about 20 feet above the road around the reservoir. Quickly other lights swiveled and focused on the same area.

"Let's go," Pam and I said simultaneously.

Pam yelled to Sam to stay on the bridge in case we wanted to move the ambulance to the road around the reservoir. As we ran past the police car, she also told Tom, who was still administering psychological first aid to Scotty in the police car, where we were going.

"I want to help," Scotty cried as he heard the sudden chaos. "I want to help find my father."

"They have all the help they need," Tom reassured him. "They'll find him soon, I'm sure. I'll stay with you until they do."

"But I want to help. Where's my dad?" he kept asking.

"We don't know yet," Tom replied. "We have to be patient."

Pam and I were both wearing sneakers, but with little thought to our footwear we ran down the parkway to a point where we could jump the protective cable fence. Once on the slope, we heedlessly started down the embankment through the snow.

I must admit, at this point, that I'm a couch potato. My children tease that I would drive to the mailbox if I could, and I consider a hike in the woods pure torture. My brother maintains that I view the outdoors as a necessary evil that one must go through to get from one inside to another.

And he's right. That's exactly how I feel. But none of this mattered then. I took one route and Pam took another as, flashlights in hand, we galloped down the steep slope. With each step, we had to lift our feet high enough to clear the snow and break its frozen crust.

In the darkness I couldn't see my feet or where I was going. I had no faith in my footing or in my ability to keep from falling. As I climbed over a fallen tree, I pictured myself lying in a heap at the foot of the slope, mangled and broken. *At least the ambulance is already here,* I thought.

Then I saw the dark lump and ran over. "He's here," I yelled as I reached the man, his body about 20 feet from the foot of the embankment. He was prevented from rolling further by a large tree and a patch of winter-bare underbrush, and he was supported about a foot off the ground by the branch mass.

He was at a strange angle, arms and legs akimbo, head thrown back and to the side. Sure that he was dead, I bent over to get my face near enough to his to check for breathing. To my amazement, although he wasn't moving his limbs, he was struggling to breathe and groaning softly with each breath. He had blood all over his face, coming, I thought, from inside of his mouth.

"He's alive," I screamed to anyone who could hear. "Tell his son."

Pam arrived beside me. "It's a minor miracle," she said. "The branches must have broken his fall."

"Yeah, but his airway is lousy and he's barely breathing. I'll take his head." Our first priority was to gain control of the man's airway. I climbed around so that I was behind his head, pulled off my heavy wool gloves, and placed one hand on each side of his head. As I pulled slight traction and straightened his head, I could feel his freezing face and I could see that his cheeks were ashen and his eyes were closed.

When I carefully aligned the man's neck and used a slight jaw thrust to open his airway, I thought I felt his breathing ease a bit. Thankfully, his breathing didn't worsen when I slowly released his jaw. Without releasing my support of the man's head, I used my fingers to examine as much of his scalp as I could reach. Miraculously, there seemed to be no obvious head injury.

I opened the man's mouth with my thumb and found that it was filled with blood and broken teeth. My first priority was to keep him from aspirating any of the material as he breathed. I swept as much of the debris as I could from his mouth, glad that I had thought to put on latex gloves beneath my winter ones.

While I dealt with the patient's head, Pam yelled, "Bring the ambulance around on the fire road and get us a trauma bag ASAP [as soon as possible]. Oxygen collars and . . . I don't know what else yet."

"Suction," I added. He had a mouth full of blood, vomit, and pieces of teeth. I bent down and whispered into the man's ear. "We're here now and we're going to help you. It is most important that you don't move." His groaning subsided, so I continued, "Can you hear me?" He groaned. "That's good. Just try to stay calm and let us take care of you." Tiny tendrils of vapor drifted up from damp spots on his inert body. I hoped the dampness wasn't caused by severe bleeding.

I saw Pete Williamson appear between a rock outcrop and the tree we were up against, his personal crash kit in hand. "Can I help?" he said.

"Are we glad to see you," Pam and I said together. I leaned over the injured man's face and said, "The Lone Ranger has arrived. Pete's a paramedic who rides with us when he's not riding on his medic rig. If I'm ever in an accident, I'd like to have him there with me."

"I jumped the call," Pete said, an apologetic smile on his face. He had responded on his own without being dispatched.

"Thank God you did."

"Is he conscious?" Pete asked.

"Not very," I answered, glad for Pete's paramedic skills. Since we are only an EMT corps, he's not allowed to do anything we can't, but his experience would prove invaluable. As a professional, he's encountered severe trauma many more times than we have.

"Can you find out what hurts, Joan?" Pete asked.

"Sir, can you tell me where it hurts?" I listened for a moment, then looked at Pete and shook my head.

"We need blankets," Pete yelled to the police and firefighters below. "And we'll need ropes." A fireman in full turnout gear and carrying a length of hose climbed up the slope, around us and up another six feet. He wrapped the hose around a tree and tied it off. Now there was something to hold on to as people clambered up and down the embankment.

Another fireman climbed up with an armload of blankets and an oxygen cylinder. Quickly, Pam set up the cylinder and put the non-rebreather mask on the man's face.

Pete opened the man's jacket and cut up the front of his sweater and shirt. "I'd like to leave the jacket on him and try to work around it," Pete said, talking both to us and to himself. "Number one, it's down and we don't need loose feathers. Number two, it's damn cold out here."

"Pam," I said, "check the wet spots. I can see steam rising from them, and they might be caused by serious bleeding."

Pam nodded and surveyed the rest of the man's body. "Lots of large abrasions and a few lacerations, but nothing life threatening. I found a closed tib-fib on his right and, from what I could feel, I think his left, too. There should be much more, but his heavy clothes must have helped cushion his fall." The lower bones—tibula and fibula—of at least one leg were broken, I thought. The man was unbelievably lucky that there was no more serious injury.

When Pete had exposed the man's chest, he said, "He's got a flail chest and I'll have to stabilize it. Pam, get a bulky dressing from the crash bag." A flail chest occurs when a broken segment of ribs moves in opposition to the rest of the rib cage. Stabilizing it would ease his breathing.

Pam handed Pete two large dressings, folded into a four-by-eight-inch pad and a roll of wide adhesive tape. He arranged the dressing over the flail segment and taped it in place.

I could feel my patient's breathing become easier. "Better," I said to Pete, "but I'm still having trouble with his airway. I need suction. Got a portable in your kit?"

Pete nodded, reached into his crash kit, and pulled out a large, bulb-type turkey baster. In addition to our fancy, portable suction units, we carry one of the giant eye droppers in each crash kit on the rig for times when we need quick airway maintenance. I was delighted that Pete also carried one in his own kit.

He opened the man's mouth and used the baster to suck out much of the blood and more of the tooth fragments that were filling his mouth.

"That's great," I said. While Pete worked, I slipped my fingers down so I could feel my patient's carotid pulse. I counted his pulse and respirations as best I could. "Pulse is about one hundred and twenty and thready, breathing twenty-eight and shallow."

"Sir, can you tell me what hurts?" Maybe the patient could respond now that he was breathing more easily.

"Back," he groaned.

"He's talking to me," I said to the crew. "Says he has pain in his back." I saw Pam squeeze the toes on his left foot through his sneaker. "Can you feel Pam touching you?" I asked.

When he was silent, I said, "I get no response."

Pam squeezed his other foot. "How about that?" I asked.

"Uhhhh," he groaned. I had no idea whether that meant that he could feel anything or not. I looked at Pam and shrugged. "Can you palpate his spine?"

Pam slid her hand under the back of his down jacket. "Several areas of abrasions and some deformity in the thoracic spine."

We had to get him down this embankment, but we also had to prevent any additional trauma to his spinal cord. The way we handled him now could mean the difference between eventual recovery and permanent paralysis.

"What's your name?" I asked.

"Ted," he whispered.

"Okay, Ted. You're doing good, and I'm right here with you all the way."

"Son?" he said.

"If that's the boy who was with you, he's fine. He's with one of our people in a warm police car." I felt the man relax a bit.

Pete placed the diaphragm of his stethoscope against the man's right upper chest. "Joan, can you ask him to take a breath?"

"Ted, take a deep breath for us." The man took a breath and Pete moved the stethoscope to the upper left. "Another," I said and as he drew another breath I could feel myself breathing with him, trying to help.

"Left lung sounds diminished. Possible pneumothorax." Pete then examined Ted's abdomen finding extreme tenderness in the upper right quadrant. "Probable internal injuries, possible liver. Let's get him out of here fast."

We heard, then saw, Sam scramble around the rock outcrop next to the tree. He was carrying collars, straps and a slatted, rollable stretcher. "I brought the Reeves. I thought it might work better than a longboard."

"Might just," Pete said. "We can slide him onto it the long way with as little spinal movement as possible." Pete reached over and again used the turkey baster to clear fluid from Ted's mouth.

"He's shivering," I said. "We've got to keep him warm. Pete, use my hat." I'm not very good in the cold, so in the winter I abandon vanity and wear an ugly, navy-blue knit cap. I was the only one wearing a hat, and Ted needed it more than I did.

Pete complied and placed the hat over Ted's head. I was worried that my own shivering might move the patient's head, so I moved and supported my elbows on my thighs.

Pam selected a "tall" cervical collar and fastened it around the man's neck. Suddenly, we heard a loud yell from the top of the embankment. "Dad! Are you okay?" I looked up and saw a face leaning over the parkway railing.

I felt the man try to get enough strength to speak. "I'll tell him," I said softly, then yelled, "He's here with us and we're taking good care of him." Then I added, "He wants you to stay where it's warm, so go back to the police car."

"I want to come down."

I saw Tom next to the boy. "Listen. Don't give your dad anything more to worry about. Stay with Tom!"

"I love you, Dad." The head disappeared.

I heard men climbing the hill and saw firefighters fastening more ropes to the trees around us. Thinking about having to climb down the slope, I tried to wiggle my toes. God, I thought, my feet are freezing.

Sam, Pete, and one of the firefighters supported the Reeves by its handles while, with me holding his head, Pam and two other firefighters slid Ted onto the stretcher. I paid careful attention as we moved him, worried about his spine. Any twisting would increase his chances of paralysis. I also knew that we were causing him a great deal of pain even though he was not conscious enough to scream. We had to keep Ted on oxygen so we placed the oxygen cylinder, padded with two heavy blankets, between his legs and strapped his entire body into the Reeves.

"The worst is over," I told Ted, now rolled in the slatted canvas the way Cleopatra was rolled in the carpet to be given to Caesar. We padded his head with two folded towels so I could let go, leaving my hat on him. "We'll carry you down from here," I said, "then I'll be back with you." I stood up, cramped and shivering.

Sam, Pete, and Pam tied ropes to the handles of the Reeves and, with the help of several firefighters, the four of us guided it down the embankment. As I walked, my feet tingled and burned inside my soaked sneakers, and I shivered. "I hope they have the heat in the back of the rig cranked up high," I muttered. "For all of us."

We were all giddy with relief when we reached the bottom of the hill. "Let's leave him on the Reeves and put the whole thing on the stretcher," I suggested.

I pulled all the linen off the stretcher and the firefighters put the Reeves, now covered with dirt, snow and debris, onto the stretcher and lifted it into the rig. As Pete, Pam, and I climbed in, we were blasted with heat. "I don't think I'll be warm for at least an hour," Pam said.

A state trooper leaned into the rig and spoke to me briefly. Then Sam started to close the back doors. "St. Luke's. Code 3?" he asked.

"Lights and siren all the way," Pete said, "but let me get a set of vitals first." Quickly, we split the seam of his right jacket sleeve, using silver duct tape to keep the feathers under control.

While Pam switched Ted to our on-board oxygen and suctioned his mouth again, Pete wrapped the BP cuff around his upper arm. With his fingers on the man's radial pulse, he inflated and then slowly deflated the cuff. "BP ninety by palp, pulse still about one hundred and twenty."

I had been watching Ted's chest rise and fall. "His breathing is thirty-two and shallow." He was breathing so quickly that he wasn't exchanging sufficient air in his lower lungs. I looked at Pam. "We may have to bag him."

"His color is okay so far," she said, adjusting the non-rebreather face mask and raising the flow level to 15 liters per minute, "and the bleeding in his mouth has stopped. I'll watch carefully." She turned and called to Sam, now in the driver's seat. "Let's move!"

About halfway to the hospital, Sam tuned the radio to the hospital frequency and Pete pressed the St. Luke's code into the keypad.

"45–01 to St. Luke's ER."

After a moment, we heard, "St. Luke's on. Go ahead 45–01."

"We are en route to your location with a victim of a fall of about seventy feet down an embankment. He has absent breath sounds on the left below a stabilized flail chest, tenderness in the upper right abdominal quadrant, spinal abrasions, and contusions. He also has probable bilateral tib-fib. Patient is currently unresponsive so neuros are unknown." Pete recited Ted's vitals. "ETA about five minutes."

"10–4, 45–01. We'll be ready for you. St. Luke's clear."

"45–01 clear."

Pete replaced the handset in its holder and said, "Let's try to get neuros."

Pam looked at me. "What's his name?"

"Ted."

Pam leaned close to Ted's ear. "Ted. Can you open your eyes?" Ted groaned and slowly opened his eyes.

"That's great. Now," she took a deep breath, "can you move your toes. Either foot."

I held my fingers against the tops of Ted's sneakers, hoping that I would feel some movement. I felt a flutter. "Yeah," I said. The toes on both feet moved. "All right!"

"Can I switch places with you?" I asked Pam. Quickly we exchanged places so I was at Ted's head. "Ted," I said to him, leaning close so he could hear me over the wail of the siren. "Your son is fine. He's with the state police who'll bring him to the hospital with your wife. I talked to the trooper just before we left the scene and he'll take good care of him."

"How . . ."

"He's fine. He wasn't hurt in the accident at all. He's one brave kid, you know. He wanted to help us look for you, but we kept him warm and safe." I didn't know how much Ted could understand, but I hoped that the sound of my voice would be reassuring.

"Thanks," he whispered. "Love them."

When we arrived at St. Luke's and unloaded our patient, they were ready for us. Before we put new linen on the stretcher and finished our paperwork, Ted was on his way to X-ray, and an operating room was already on standby.

As we walked back to the rig, ready to return to Fairfax, I glanced into the waiting room and saw Scotty clinging to a woman who I assumed must be his mother. "Hi, Scotty," I said, walking toward him. "I don't know whether you saw me earlier, but I was at the accident."

"How's my dad?"

"I was with him all the time. He's holding his own and the hospital is taking super care of him. In the ambulance, he asked me to tell you both that he loves you."

The woman reached out and squeezed my hand. "Thank you for everything."

Two days later I called the hospital and asked for Ted's floor. "Ted is in stable condition," the floor nurse told me. "He spent considerable time in surgery, but they were able to repair his lacerated liver. He has bilateral lower-leg fractures, but they're healing nicely. The punctured lung will heal itself."

"Any sign of spinal injury?" I asked.

"Some bruising and swelling, but the neurologist doesn't expect any permanent impairment."

"Yeah," I said. "All right!"

"Excuse me?"

"Nothing. Thanks so much for the report. And be good to him."

NAVIGATING AROUND TOWN

WHEN I FIRST joined the ambulance corps, I thought that an ambulance was an esoteric machine that required deep understanding to drive. I remember my shock when, for the first time, I was in the rig when we stopped for gas. You fill it up just like a car, I thought. How amazing. Then I took my driver-training course and learned that each of our rigs is simply a small, six-wheeled truck body with a "box" on the back that is the ambulance itself.

When I first became a driver, my younger daughter, not yet a member of the corps, teased me unmercifully. "Mom," she said, "you get lost on your way to the mailbox."

"They have a Rolodex at headquarters," I explained, "with a card in it for each street in town and precise directions that even I can follow."

Now when I respond from home, I still frequently need to have the police give me precise instructions, even to some of the more common locations. But from headquarters, navigation is easy. I grab the card and go.

Unfortunately, because most of the calls I respond to are at night, I have another problem with directions. A few of the young people in town have recently made a game of collecting the town's new, bright blue and white street signs. Frequently, I have to backtrack or count intersections trying to follow what should be simple directions.

Because I am sometimes the first one at the scene in the middle of the night, finding the right street is no guarantee of being able to find the house. Many houses in Fairfax have no numbers, either on the house or on the mailbox. When the police talk to the caller, they request that someone turn on a front light so that we will know when we've found the right house. Occasionally, however, in the heat of the moment, people forget. It can be very frustrating to have to radio the police and have them call the victim's family back while I sit in my idling car knowing that I could be helping a patient.

ADAPTATION

MEMBERS WHO TAKE as many day calls as Ed and I do have changed their ways of doing everyday things.

Because many calls require trips through long grass where deer ticks are common, and through poison ivy, brambles, and rose thorns, I keep my lower body protected at all times. I almost always wear long pants, even in the heat of the summer, and I never wear sandals. I never wear sweatpants, because they have no pockets on which to clip my radio. (I've tried to clip the heavy transmitter to an elastic waistband, but I must admit that every time I do, the pants slip down past my hips.)

Because we're not always in uniform when we respond to ambulance calls, Ed and I usually wear corps-approved navy-blue jackets. We each have both a light, summer-weight windbreaker and a heavy, fleece-lined winter jacket, all with the "star of life" logo on the back, a patch that identifies us as members of FVAC, and a state EMT patch on the sleeve. The corps also has hooded yellow raincoats with the same logo on the back in reflective blue, for nights and bad weather. Occasionally, when we're responding from home, we'll ask the driver to bring extra rain jackets for us.

I carry latex gloves everywhere, in all my pockets, in my pocketbook, and in the glove compartment of my car. I always put gloves on, either on the way to the call or right before I step out of my car.

Recently, I treated myself to a man-sized new watch with a white face, large black numerals, and an easy-to-see sweep secondhand, which I wear every day. I can take a pulse and respiration or check times for the PCR without having to put my glasses on.

Ed and I both carry crash kits in our trunks. Ed's is an old backpack and mine is a Rubbermaid toolbox. A typical crash kit contains a few pairs of latex gloves and enough large and small square sterile pads and roller gauze, triangular bandages, and chemical ice packs to attend to a patient until a rig arrives. Also in our kits we carry a BP cuff and a stethoscope for taking vitals, a pad and pen for recording them, and a quarter for phoning for help if necessary.

In our state, a flashing green emergency light identifies a member of an ambulance corps, while a blue one identifies a member of a volunteer fire department or rescue squad. Many volunteers have had lights permanently mounted; Ed's light stays magnetically attached to the roof of his car at all times.

Kojak lights are very useful, but I've always been amazed by the ease with which unmarked police cars in the movies position them. They open the driver's side window, reach out through it and plop the light on the roof. Then they are able to get out of the driver's door without removing the light. I wonder how they manage that, with the top of the window frame now tangled in the coils of the light cord? That's Hollywood, I guess.

As trained professionals, EMTs may assist accident or illness victims at any time or place. I have come to the aid of patients in the New York City subway system, in high-rise office buildings, and on many roads outside of my own ambulance district. Ed has responded in similar situations, as well as to emergencies involving his own family members and, in one case, a dog.

We have even cared for the victim of a bloody swimming accident on a nude beach in the Caribbean. It gave new meaning to the lesson we teach, that an EMT must be prepared to use whatever is available.

FOUR

THERE ARE FEW situations guaranteed to produce as many conflicting feelings in an EMT as a call that involves assisting an emotionally disturbed person (EDP). This can be anyone from a person who has temporarily freaked out, stoned on some drug, to a person who is a diagnosed psychotic or a habitual alcoholic.

This type of patient is usually unpredictable, sometimes violent, occasionally helpless, and often deserving of our sympathy. The calls are usually frustrating, because, our emergency medical training is often useless in these situations. We must rely only on whatever person-to-person communication skills we have developed. And sometimes these calls are dangerous.

Music was blasting at decibel levels that rivaled those produced by 747 jet engines during takeoff; we could hear it all the way down the hundred-foot-long, treelined driveway.

"Holy shit, Ed. I've never seen anything like this except in *Lifestyles of the Rich and Famous*." Nick Abrams was not usually impressed by material things, but this house was beyond description. Although it was late evening and fully dark, the front of the house was ablaze with enough light to land aircraft.

"This is some mansion," I responded, gazing at the manicured lawn and carefully pruned shrubbery. "Must've gone for a million anyway. I bet there's a pool, tennis courts, the works." We all knew that Whitehouse Road contains estates that range in size from four to 30 acres, and this one appeared to be one of the biggest.

Light blazed from every window in the three-story colonial, and the front of the house was littered with Mercedeses, Rollses, Jaguars, and an occasional classic BMW. "The dispatcher said we have an unconscious male. Maybe he got run over by his yacht," Sam Middleton mumbled.

"Or maybe we'll have to fish him out of his hot tub," Nick said.

No one heard us knock or ring the doorbell, so we pushed the front door open and walked in. The air in the huge living room was filled with a thick, smoky haze, one breath of which explained the glassy-eyed look of most of the teenagers in the room. I wondered how long our rescue crew could remain in this atmosphere without getting a contact high ourselves.

While much of the group gyrated to the rhythm of the blaring music, others were draped on the furniture in various states of undress. No one seemed to notice the appearance of the three uniformed party-crashers or even seemed to be aware of any medical emergency. Then, in a corner of the room, we saw a young man of about eighteen waving to us. He was well-groomed, clean shaven, and he had a diamond stud in one ear. He was wearing designer jeans, a pink shirt with a prestigious emblem on the pocket, and snakeskin loafers.

We made our way through the mob of dancing kids, and the pink-shirted young man motioned toward another boy of about fifteen or sixteen, lying faceup on the floor, eyes closed. He looked peaceful, seemingly uninjured. He was small, about five feet four, and slight, no more than 120 pounds. He had bright red hair and was dressed in brown leather pants, a black suede jacket, and a light blue open-necked shirt. His face was slightly flushed, and he was barefoot.

"Is he breathing?" I yelled as I arrived at the boy's side.

"Don't know," the boy said.

I knelt down next to the redheaded youth and put my ear near his face, looking down toward his chest. Although the noise in the room precluded my hearing anything, I could feel his breath on my cheek and could see his chest rise and fall.

"Are you okay?" I yelled, but the boy didn't move. "Wake up. Wake up!" I took the knuckle of my index finger and ground it into the boy's breastbone. There was no reaction to what normally would have been a painful sternal rub.

I looked at the boy who had beckoned us over. "What happened?"

"I don't know," he replied. "He just went out."

"What is he on?" I asked.

"Nothing. Not a thing," the boy answered defensively. "We don't do drugs or any of that shit."

Chuck Harding, the Fairfax policeman who had followed us in, tried to talk to him. "Look, I'm not going to bust you. We just need to know what your friend is on so we can help him. What is it? Pot? Crack? What?"

"Not a fuckin' thing," the boy repeated, backing away. Then he turned and disappeared into the mass of gyrating teenagers.

Realizing that we were going to get no help from the other kids, I examined the boy's head while Sam went over his arms and chest and Nick surveyed his lower body. Chuck pulled the boy's wallet from his jacket pocket.

"Anything?" I asked.

"Not a thing," the two other EMTs said.

"I found his driver's license," Chuck said.

We took a quick set of vitals and found that his pulse was rapid, his breathing shallow, and his blood pressure a bit low. I pulled up his upper eyelid and saw that his pupils were dilated.

No one in the room paid any attention to us as we put the boy on high-flow oxygen and lifted his limp body onto a stretcher. We loaded him into the ambulance and began our trip to Fairfax General Hospital, code 3.

The trip to Fairfax General was uneventful. Although he appeared to be in a deep state of unconsciousness, the boy's vital signs remained stable. At the hospital, we wheeled him into the ER and, by bunching up and grasping the sides of the stretcher sheet and pulling, we slid him onto the ER examination table with as little movement to his body as possible.

While the rest of the crew rolled the stretcher into the ER anteroom and began to make it up with clean linen, I remained with the patient until the doctor came over.

"What have we got here?" Dr. Margolis asked.

"Not a clue. We found him unresponsive to pain. Indications of substance abuse by the condition of everyone else in the room. But no one at the scene could give us . . ."

Suddenly, the boy's eyes flew open and he shot up into a sitting position. Wild-eyed, he looked down at his feet, then turned his dilated pupils toward me.

"You stole my shoes," he shrieked, his eyes boring into mine, "and I'm going to kill you."

At that moment, looking into his crazed eyes, I was sure that he could kill me. Slightly uncoordinated, the redheaded boy swung his legs over the edge of the gurney. Still glaring at me, the boy dropped his bare feet to the floor. As he stalked me, I began to back away slowly. "Fuckin' thief," he shrieked. "You stole my shoes!"

Glancing around, I realized that everyone in the room was as terrified of this kid as I was. I couldn't figure out why anyone else was worried. He seemed to have a singular purpose. Killing me.

"Quick, get into the doctor's lounge and shut the door," one of the nurses whispered to me as she reached under an instrument shelf to press the button that would summon security guards.

I needed no urging. I turned and sprinted the few feet to the doctor's lounge adjacent to the boy's cubicle. I slammed the door and, because there was no lock, leaned against it. For some reason, instead of trying the knob, the boy launched himself against the door. I heard and felt, first the boy's shoulder, then his fists pound on the wood. Fortunately it held. The pounding sound was then replaced by the sound of running and a series of crashes. The red-haired boy, who had been sleeping so peacefully only moments before, was back in the ER cubicle, bent on destruction.

There was a small, curtained window in the wall between the lounge and the cubicle. Hesitantly curious, I waited a minute to be sure the boy wasn't coming back, then lifted the corner of the drape and peeked out.

The scene was complete chaos. Having been denied his wish to kill me, the boy was systematically demolishing everything he could reach. Linen, metal basins, first aid supplies, everything within his reach was now scattered around the cubicle area. A six-foot-three, 250 pound security guard who had tried to stop him was now lying in a heap in the corner, groggily rubbing his left temple.

The boy stood, his back toward me, with a clear plastic bag of IV solution in each hand. As I watched, he hurled them at the wall. "Shit, shit, shit," he screamed, seemingly disappointed that the plastic containers remained undamaged. He ran across the room and stomped on one of the containers with the heel of one bare foot. He seemed pleased when the container burst, spraying sterile saline over the wreckage in the room. Wild-eyed, he looked around the floor for the other plastic bag. I heaved a sigh. At least he seemed to have forgotten about killing me.

After what felt like an eternity, I heard the sound of sirens as two state police cars pulled up in front of the hospital. Through the lounge window, I saw two troopers rush in followed by two more hefty hospital security guards. As the redheaded boy jumped up and down on the second plastic saline container, one guard grabbed his left arm in a hammerlock and the other grabbed his right. One trooper grabbed his two legs at the ankles and the other seized him at the knees. It took the four men almost a minute to wrestle the wildly struggling young man onto a gurney.

As they started to tie restraints to his wrists and ankles, the redheaded boy's body suddenly went limp as he again lapsed into a state of unconsciousness. To prevent a recurrence of his bizarre behavior, they restrained him despite his unresponsiveness. As quickly as I could, I finished my paperwork, left the ER, and rode back to headquarters.

I returned to the hospital the following morning with another patient. The ER looked normal, with no sign of last night's craziness. I saw Dr. Margolis in the hall. "Where's our patient from last night?"

"He slept for four hours, then complained that he had to pee. We let him go to the john with two security guards. He gave them the slip and disappeared."

"Ever find out what he was on?"

"We drew blood, but whatever it was is too new to be on our drug profile. People keep inventing new 'designer drugs' faster than we can keep up. We'll probably see him again."

Fervently, I said, "I hope I never do."

○ ○ ○

MOST RESCUE CALLS deal with single incidents, a car accident or a heart attack. Sometimes we are able to help our patient, sometimes not. The patient either dies or gets better. But EDPs are a never-ending source of frustration for us. They are often "regulars"—people for whom we are called repeatedly, and for whom there is little or nothing that we can do.

It began five years ago, at about three o'clock one morning, when the phone rang.

"Ed? Fairfax Police. Sorry to bother you, but you and Joan are on the duty crew and we need a rig at 370 Oak Hill Lane for an EDP. We have a unit at the scene and crisis intervention is there, too."

"Okay. Joan and I'll pick up the rig. Will you call Bob?" Bob Fiorella was the third member of our crew that night. "Ask him to meet us at the scene."

The house was in a development of identical raised ranches on a quiet street. Joan and I entered the house, followed closely by Bob, who had arrived just behind the rig. We were met at the door by Stan Poritsky, a Fairfax Police Officer, who looked totally bewildered.

"What's up?" I asked.

"I hope you can sort it out. It's chaos here."

We walked up the half flight of carpeted stairs and into a small, comfortably furnished living room. At one end of the sofa, a scruffy-looking woman was deep in conversation with an older man. An obviously pregnant woman, curled in the fetal position was deep in thought at the other end. A man stood in the center of the room, chanting, "Michelle has to go. She doesn't want to go, but we all know that she has to go."

"I hate dealing with EDPs," Bob muttered.

"I couldn't agree more," I said.

"Michelle has to go," the man intoned again. "She doesn't want to go, but we all know that she has to go."

"Where is crisis intervention?" I asked Stan who had followed us up the stairs. "I thought they had been called."

Stan pointed toward the couch. When I still looked baffled, he said, "You obviously haven't met Dr. Cardone. She's head of the Oakside Psychiatric Hospital's crisis intervention team. Over there talking to that man." Stan pointed to the hawk-nosed woman in her early forties, sitting on the sofa and talking heatedly with a nicely dressed older man. Dr. Cardone turned, as if she had heard her name, although how she could have heard anything over the chanting, I didn't know.

Dr. Cardone's platinum crew cut was only about one inch long all over her head. She wore a kelly green sweatshirt with a beer logo on the front, green sweatpants, and sandals. A silver ankh dangled from her right ear. She held a small leather case in one hand and a cigarette in the other.

We edged around the man in the center of the room and crouched in front of Dr. Cardone. "I'm glad you're here," she said, waving her cigarette in my face. She momentarily stopped her conversation and pointed to the pregnant woman, sitting silently, hugging her enlarged belly. "She's got to go to the hospital. It's the best thing for her."

"What is her problem . . . doctor?" I asked. Because of her totally un-doctorlike appearance, I found it hard to use her title.

"She is worried about her unborn baby, and that upsets everyone else." Dr. Cardone pointed to the man, still singing. "When Larry, her husband, called me, I came right over. I've been treating Michelle for a long time. She's a very disturbed person."

I could almost feel Michelle curl up tighter.

"Michelle has to go. She doesn't want to go, but we all know that she has to go."

Dr. Cardone, her back still to Michelle, said, "You'll probably have to restrain her. She doesn't want to go to the hospital, but I know what's best for her. She's been there several times before."

I turned and saw that tears now slipped quietly down Michelle's cheeks. "We'll be right back," I told Dr. Cardone, leading Joan and Bob out of the room.

Bob had a very strong opinion on how to handle the situation. "I think that we should restrain the psychiatrist and the woman's husband and take them both to the loony bin. They're obviously the crazy ones." From the look on Bob's face, it was apparent that he wasn't joking entirely. "We have no authority to restrain and forcibly transport that woman," he continued, "and besides, she's not a threat to anyone. Let's tell her to stick it in her ear."

"Has anyone talked to the patient?" Joan suggested. "Cardone's a little strange, but it seems to me that Michelle would be better off out of here. She looks totally lost. And Oakside is a good psychiatric facility." Joan looked at me. "Let me see if I can get her to come with us voluntarily."

"You're welcome to try," I said. Joan's unusually good with people, and having Michelle agree to be transported would solve our whole problem.

Joan walked back to the sofa and crouched next to Michelle while I stood quietly behind. The woman wore no makeup, so her pallor and the deep circles under her eyes were obvious.

"My name's Joan," she began. "Dr. Cardone thinks you'd be better off out of here. Would you like to come with us?"

Tears fell from Michelle's eyes. Joan slowly reached out her hand. "Would you like to hold my hand? I'm good at hand-holding."

For the first time, Michelle made eye contact. Lightly, Joan placed her fingertips on the back of one of Michelle's hands, still resting on her belly. "We're not going to hold you down or hurt you, Michelle," Joan said. "But we might be able to help."

Michelle shook her head slowly but didn't pull her hand away from Joan's fingers.

"I see you're quite pregnant. How soon is the baby due?"

Michelle slowly raised two fingers. "Two months?" Joan asked. Michelle nodded.

"I have two children myself," Joan said, "both girls. But they're both grown and moved away. You look like you could use some sleep, and I'll bet it's not easy to get any rest with that big belly in your way."

"Can I walk?"

"You mean to the ambulance? Of course you can walk, if you like. Okay?"

She nodded, and I was delighted. With her now agreeing, I just wanted to get her out of there as quickly as I could.

"Would you like someone to get your coat? It's a bit chilly outside."

The man in the center of the room had quieted but now began again. "She's gonna go. She's gonna go."

"Coat's downstairs," Michelle mumbled.

Awkwardly, Michelle rose and, with amazing poise, walked down the stairs. Without another word, she retrieved her coat and walked to the ambulance.

We helped her through the back doors and sat her on the crew bench. Joan sat down next to her and buckled Michelle's seat belt. "Would you like to hold my hand?" she asked.

Again Michelle nodded. She didn't speak again during the long ride to Oakside and, when we arrived, she quietly left the rig and walked with us into the lobby.

"Thanks," she said as she went through the heavy double doors and out of our sight.

"You're welcome," we said, happy that a bad situation had ended, at least for the moment.

Unhappily, hospitals, crisis intervention teams, and ambulance volunteers were unable to help Michelle very much. Over the next five years she became one of our "regulars," and I returned to her house several times. The crew and I were usually met by Dr. Cardone, who frequently advised restraints to force her to get treatment. We were always able to convince her to come without them.

As time passed, I watched Michelle become increasingly disturbed and despondent and in the last two years, addicted to alcohol. We were called more and more often to transport her to the hospital or to a detoxification center.

Then, one day I saw the following brief item in the local newspaper:

"Woman, thirty-nine, found dead in state park in Fairfax."

The story went on. "The woman, Michelle Morris, of Oak Hill Lane, Fairfax, was found by joggers shortly before eight o'clock last Tuesday morning. She was lying on her side in the snow about half a mile from her home, dressed only in a short-sleeved polo shirt and jeans.

"The cause of death is tentatively listed as exposure. She was married and the mother of two, the police said."

I found myself weeping, as much for our own limitations as for Michelle.

○ ○ ○

EMERGENCY MEDICAL WORK does not always involve immediate and fast action. Often we are called upon to stand by at potentially dangerous situations such as scenes of fires, bomb threats, suicide threats, and occasionally, hostage situations—just in case.

It was about 7 P.M. in early September. We had checked out the rigs and were about to begin dinner. Our shift had been quiet for the last few weeks.

"There's a full moon tonight," Jack said, looking up from the TV set. "We'll probably get a call."

Jack McCaffrey was a professor at Fairfax Community College, a very quiet and usually very rational man.

"Yeah," Linda replied. "We're always extra busy in the ER when there's a full moon out."

Linda Potemski had been an emergency room nurse for 20 years and a member of the Fairfax Ambulance Corps for 15 years. She was a thoroughly competent nurse and EMT.

I am always amazed that otherwise rational people can believe in the ability of a full moon to cause emergency situations to occur. Yet almost every police officer, EMT, or ER nurse who I know swears that they are busier on full-moon nights. And despite the fact that every study has shown no increase in crimes, suicides, or any other human behavior on the night of the full moon, I sometimes believe it myself. There is something in the nature of emergency work—the capriciousness, unpredictability, and uncontrollability of it, the fact that we can be calmly having dinner one moment and racing to the scene of a life-and-death situation the next—that makes many emergency workers superstitious. Our world often seems turned upon a throw of dice by the gods.

"639 to 312," the scanner droned. The police were calling one of their cars.

"312 on." I recognized Will McAndrews's voice.

"Are you aware of the situation?"

"Yeah, affirmative."

"Detective Greenberg would like you to respond to the scene."

"10–4. Is he there yet?"

"Affirmative."

"I'm en route," the voice on the scanner answered.

Normally, the chatter on our headquarters scanner is only a background sound. There is constant police and fire communication and dispatches from county control, but we usually ignore it unless something is said that is relevant to us. We tune in only when we hear terms such as 10–2: a personal injury automobile accident; 10–3: an emergency medical situation, or something unusual.

"I wonder what's going on?" Linda said.

Tonight something was going on that the police did not want to broadcast. From the nature of the cryptic messages it was obvious that most of the communications were being broadcast on the alternate police channel—the private channel to which we had no access. But the fact that a detective was responding meant that something serious was going on.

"639 to 308."

"Go ahead."

"Crisis intervention ETA is approximately ten minutes."

"10–4."

"Something's sure happening," I said to Jack and Linda. "I don't know about that full moon stuff, but I have a funny feeling we're not going to get to finish our dinner."

As if on cue, the telephone rang. I lifted the receiver. "Fairfax Ambulance, Ed Herman speaking."

"Hi, Ed. It's Mark Thomas at police headquarters. We didn't want to put this out over the radio, but we need you to respond with an ambulance for a standby at 844 Franklin Street. Try to be as quiet as possible; no lights or siren. Park around the corner on Jackson. You'll see a number of patrol cars there."

"What've you got, Mark?" I asked.

"We have a sixty-five-year-old man who's holding a sawed-off shotgun to his head and threatening suicide. The guy's name is Sam Whitley. His son lives in California and his wife died a few weeks ago. He's all alone and obviously very despondent. We have him on the phone, trying to get him to allow someone to come in to talk to him, but he says he'll blow his own head off if anyone tries to enter the house."

"Okay. We'll respond nice and easy," I assured him, then hung up. "Let's go," I said to the crew. "We've got a suicide standby at Franklin and Jackson."

"Aw, shit," Jack and Linda said in unison, looking down wistfully at their unfinished dinners.

We got into the ambulance, quietly drove to Jackson Street, and parked behind three darkened patrol cars.

At around 10 P.M., one of the officers brought us sandwiches and coffee. We ate, then continued to wait for something to happen.

At about 1 A.M., Dr. Cardone, the head of the crisis intervention team, finally entered the house. Earlier, she had convinced Sam to allow her to come into the house, but Sam had insisted that she come in alone—no cops. At first the police had refused to allow Dr. Cardone to go in alone. The man was armed and, even though he had threatened only himself, they could not guarantee the doctor's safety. But after a three-hour stalemate, the police had reluctantly agreed.

By 3:30 in the morning, our adrenaline rushes had long worn off. Linda was asleep on the stretcher, and Jack on the crew bench in the back of the rig. I was trying to make myself comfortable in the cab with little success. It was starting to get chilly in the ambulance and I considered closing the windows, but I loved listening to the symphony of sound in the late-summer night. There was always music outside at this time of the year. Cicadas during the day and a chorus of crickets and katydids at night. For me, life seemed so rich and joyous. For the man in the house, life must be so bleak, I thought.

Cardone had been talking to Sam for hours, and I wondered how much longer we would be stuck here. I was tired, hungry, and bored. Suddenly the insect-song-filled silence of the night was shattered by the sound of an explosion. Instantly, running figures converged upon the house.

"What's going on?" Linda asked, her voice still thick with sleep.

"I don't know," I answered. "That sounded more like a bomb than a gunshot."

We were all awake now, waiting for the police to call us in. A minute went by. Two minutes. Our protocol was to sit tight until the police called for us.

Three minutes went by, and I opened the ambulance door. "I can't just stay here any longer," I said. "I'm going to see what's going on."

I got out of the rig, walked around the corner, and approached the small ranch-style house. Through the living room window I could see policemen and civilians, who I assumed were members of the crisis team, moving around slowly. At the front door, detective Irv Greenberg was talking to a uniformed officer. I walked up to the front door.

"Are you going to need us, Irv?" I asked.

He glanced at me. "Oh, sorry, Ed. I forgot that you guys were around the corner waiting." He hesitated, as if not knowing what to say. "You can go in and examine him if you want to, but there's not much point to it. Cardone couldn't talk him down, and he finally did it. Most of his head is gone."

I sighed and said, "If you say he's beyond our help, we'll go home now."

If there had been any doubt about the condition of the patient, I would have insisted on examining him myself. But I was willing to take Irv's word that a patient with most of his head blown away was dead. And I most definitely did not want to see him if I didn't have to.

I pulled my portable out of its holster and keyed the mike to call the rig. "45–01 portable to 45–01."

"45–01 on," Linda answered.

"We're released from standby. Let's go home."

"10–4," the radio crackled.

○ ○ ○

FAIRFAX IS A NIMBY(not in my backyard) town. Most of the citizens of Fairfax have emigrated from The Big City, seeking quiet treelined streets, well-kept lawns, and two-car garages. They moved to Fairfax to escape the problems of the city, and they don't want to be reminded of these problems.

Whenever there has been an attempt to set up a group home for the mentally, emotionally, or physically disabled in Fairfax, it has been vigorously opposed on the grounds that "we have enough group homes." I have never been able to learn what the criteria are for deciding how many is enough.

When a national drug rehabilitation organization decided to set up a drug-recovery center for teenagers in a building located in a remote part of town, people almost took to the streets. An ad hoc group of concerned citizens ran full-page ads in the local newspaper, warning of rape, pillage, and plunder should the facility move into town. Every time such an ad appeared, I clipped it, attached a donation check, and sent it along with a note saying that not all Fairfax citizens feel that way about the center. The facility was finally set up in Fairfax about ten years ago, and the town police have had far more problems with local teenagers than they have had with the teenaged residents of the center.

It's not that the good people of Fairfax are against drug-rehabilitation centers or group homes. They just feel that they should be somewhere else—not in their backyard. Yet, despite my feeling that such facilities do belong in a town such as Fairfax, occasionally there have been ambulance calls that have made me question how well some of these facilities are managed.

It had been an unusually quiet, cold, dark winter evening when the call came in for an unknown injury at the group home on River Road. As we frequently do, we turned off our lights and siren before we pulled on to River Road to avoid further exciting a potentially disturbed person.

"45–01 on location," I reported as we pulled to a stop in the group home's driveway. The home occupied a five-bedroom house in a usually quiet neighborhood. I had been there once before and knew it to be run by a small staff. It usually housed about half a dozen residents.

"10–4," the radio answered. "Your time is 21:01."

The police had not yet arrived, there was no one outside to meet the ambulance, and the front porch was dark. We wondered whether we were in the right place, but as we stepped out of the rig, we could hear loud voices coming from the usually quiet house. Something was obviously going on.

The three of us glanced at one another and hesitated. In a dangerous situation, our protocol is to wait for the police to secure the scene before we enter. But the dispatcher hadn't indicated any danger, just that there was a medical problem.

I was riding with my daughter Davida that evening. Before joining the senior corps, she had been an FVAC youth group cadet and had responded to several calls. But she was still young and inexperienced. "Do we go in?" she asked, looking at me with a frown on her face. She trusted me, both as her father and as a senior member of the crew, to decide what to do.

Fred Stevens, our third member, was one of the corps's old-timers. He was short and heavy, and, particularly when excited, he used profanity whenever possible. But he was a good and experienced EMT.

"What the fuck do you figure's going on in there?" Fred asked.

"Beats me," I replied as I pulled the radio out of my belt. "45–01 portable to Fairfax Police."

"Go ahead 01."

"Do you have any further dispatch information?" I asked.

"Negative."

"Is there an officer en route to this location?"

"Yeah, affirmative. Officer Berkowitz should be there momentarily."

Berkowitz, I thought. He's that new guy I had met for the first time on a call a few days earlier. He looked like a young kid fresh out of high school.

"What the fuck," Fred said. "The cop'll be here soon enough. Let's see what the hell's going on."

When we received no answer to our knock on the front door, we opened it and stepped directly into a large, well-lit room. A woman who appeared to be in her mid-thirties was sitting in a chair in the center of the room clutching her right hand between her legs, tears streaming down her face. A young man in jeans and a navy-blue T-shirt was circling her, moving back and forth and stopping frequently to kick out at her, although not close enough to actually hit her.

As we approached her, the young man moved back, still circling and kicking. The four other young people in the room all appeared to be in their late teens and twenties and were very agitated; two women were pacing the length of the room while two young men sat on the floor rocking and screaming.

"Are you the one who's injured?" Fred asked the seated woman.

"Yes. I'm the evening resident-supervisor, and I think my finger is broken," she replied through clenched teeth.

"What happened?"

"Jake," she nodded toward the boy who was circling and kicking at us, "got mad at me and slammed a door on my finger."

"Are you alone here?" Davida asked.

"During the night I'm alone with our five residents. It's usually quiet, but this afternoon Jake had some trouble with his parents and wouldn't go to bed. I tried to calm him down, but obviously I had little success. Now he seems to have focused his anger on me."

"Let me see your finger," Fred requested.

The woman held her hand up. Her index finger was discolored, swollen, and deformed near the base—obviously a bad, closed fracture.

"Did he do it deliberately?" Fred asked.

"In a way, yes."

"Bastard," Fred muttered, glowering at the boy.

"No. Don't blame him," the woman said. "He's normally a pussycat. All these people are like children. None of them has a mental age above seven. They're good, loving people despite their handicap, but sometimes they get upset."

"What's your name?" Fred asked.

"Paula. Paula Gebhardt."

"Paula, I'm Fred and this is Ed and Davida." He turned as he heard someone open the front door. "And that's Merve Berkowitz." He pointed at the Fairfax policeman who was coming toward us. "Paula," Fred continued, "your finger looks like it's broken. We're going to have to put a splint on it, and then we'll take you over to Fairfax General. Okay?"

"I guess," Paula said, lowering her hand, "but I can't leave until Harriet Corbett, another resident-supervisor, gets here. I called her a little while ago, and she should be here in a few minutes."

"We'll get you splinted and hopefully she'll be here before we're ready to leave. I'll hold her hand up, Ed," Fred said. "Why don't you splint it."

"Davida," I directed after examining the injury more closely, "get me a roll of two-inch gauze." As Davida rummaged around in the crash bag, I warned Paula, "I'll do this as gently, as I can but it's probably going to hurt."

Paula nodded as Davida handed me the gauze. "I want you to keep your injured finger next to your middle finger, separate from the other fingers so I can immobilize the injured one against the other."

I gently placed the roll of gauze against her finger. Paula sucked a breath in through her teeth and whimpered as the soft gauze touched her broken finger. Fred held her hand while I began to wind the strip around the two fingers.

I had been so focused on the job of immobilizing Paula's hand with the least amount of pain that I had paid no attention to Jake who, still circling and kicking, had gradually inched closer. Suddenly Jake ran over to us, reached between Davida and me, and, before we could react, grabbed Paula's broken finger and twisted it.

The attack and Paula's agonized scream had an electrifying effect on the home's other four residents. The two young men who had been pacing began to pound on the wall and the two women were shrieking and rocking in place. Jake was kicking again, his feet ending up much closer now, almost touching us.

Officer Berkowitz, ashen-faced, grabbed his radio from its holster, keyed the mike, and yelled, "317 to 639. 10–13."

10–13—officer needs assistance. I knew that would bring almost every officer in Fairfax to the scene, lights flashing and sirens screaming.

"Merve," I said urgently, trying to act as calmly as I could, "tell them not to use their sirens. If these people get any more agitated than they already are, we're all in big trouble."

Merve nodded agreement. "317 to 639," he radioed. "Do not use sirens," he pleaded. "Repeat. Do not use sirens under any circumstances."

"10–4, 317," the dispatcher answered. "No sirens." Merve didn't want to wait for backup to arrive. The situation was getting too dangerous and was out of our control.

"Okay," Merve ordered. "We're going to move slowly and quietly toward the door as a group. I want Paula in the center in case the boy tries to attack her again. I'll bring up the rear. If any of them get too close, run for the door. I will try to hold them off until you can all get out."

As we inched toward the door, Jake continued circling and kicking, just short of making contact. I wondered whether he would attack as we approached the door, but he got no closer. At last, when Fred was able to reach out and pull open the front door, we dashed toward the ambulance just as police cars began silently converging on the scene.

Harriet Corbett arrived as we settled Paula in the ambulance, and she and a few Fairfax police officers were able to calm the residents of the home without further violence. Paula was treated and released at the hospital, and she returned to the group home before lunch.

Fortunately, events like that are rare and I'm still in favor of allowing group homes in Fairfax. But as with all of my opinions, I'm not nearly as certain as I was 20 years ago.

THE NUMBERS GAME I

IN OUR COUNTY, every ambulance corps and rescue squad has its own two-digit prefix number. As you already know, the prefix for Fairfax Ambulance is 45. For Prescott, a neighboring corps, the prefix is 21. The rigs are usually numbered from 01 on, so, for example, Fairfax's first rig is 45–01, the second is 45–02, and the third is 45–03.

Each member of the corps who has a portable two-way radio has his/her own two-digit suffix. The captain of any corps is identified by the suffix 11, the first lieutenant is 12, and the second lieutenant is 13. Others have suffixes of 20 or higher.

My call number is 45–22, and Joan's is 45–24.

The base station has an FCC-assigned combination of letters and numbers that must be used at the beginning of each transmission. Each radio transmission should end with the word "clear" or "over" so that anyone else waiting to use the same frequency knows that he can proceed with his transmission.

GKL-642 is assigned to the Fairfax Volunteer Ambulance Corps, GBY-639 to the Fairfax Police Department, and GRQ-325 to the Prescott Police Department.

THE NUMBERS GAME II

RADIO COMMUNICATION SOMETIMES becomes garbled, and for many years code numbers have been used to speed and clarify transmission. Certain of the ten codes—for example "ten-four, good buddy"—were popularized during the CB craze. For your edification, I've included a list of the most common ten codes that Fairfax Ambulance uses. Be aware, however, that other services, particularly fire departments and police, have different meanings for these numbers.

10–1—property damage auto accident
10–2—personal injury auto accident
10–3—aided case—illness or injury for causes other than an auto accident
10–4—I heard your transmission and acknowledge
10–8—back in service after a call
10–13—police code for officer needs assistance
10–17—returning to headquarters
10–42—stopping for gas
10–45—obvious death
10–99—CPR in progress

On occasion, the ten codes can lead to very cryptic conversations.

"45–01 to 642. Be advised we are 10–8 from the 10–2. We will be 10–42 then 10–17."

"10–4, 45–01. 15:25. 642 clear."

Did you understand that? During the first transmission the crew reported that the Fairfax first rig was back in service after a call for a personal injury auto accident. They then stated that they were going to stop for gas and return to headquarters.

The base dispatcher responded that he had understood the transmission from the Fairfax first rig. Then the dispatcher gave the current time, on a 24-hour clock (military time), as 3:25 in the afternoon. Times between midnight (00:00) and noon (1200 hours) are the same on the military clock as on the standard clock. Times between noon and midnight are the current clock time plus twelve hours. Therefore 3:25 P.M. is 3:25 + or 12:00 or 15:25. The base dispatcher ended the dialogue by saying that the base station was ending transmission.

THE NUMBERS GAME III

THERE ARE THREE ways to drive an ambulance.

Code 1 indicates that the ambulance is off duty or on duty but without a current call. The driver may stop for a pizza.

Code 2 indicates that the ambulance is on duty, but not responding to an emergency. It may be returning from the hospital, on a nonemergency transport call, or responding to the hospital with a patient whose condition does not require emergency driving procedures. While driving code 2, the ambulance must obey all traffic laws. When responding to an emergency, if an EMT at the scene suggests that the ambulance can "respond with caution," it may respond code 2.

Code 3 indicates that the ambulance is responding to an emergency or is being driven to the hospital with a patient in serious condition. During code 3 driving, an ambulance driver must use all emergency warning lights and sound its siren. The ambulance is then exempt from most traffic laws, but must not be driven in a reckless manner. Although the ambulance may pass through any red light, the ambulance should stop, or at least slow significantly, at all intersections and must be sure that the road is clear in every direction before proceeding.

When responding to an emergency, we rarely drive faster than the speed limit and avoid violating traffic regulations whenever possible. Yet, we cannot wait in traffic. Someone's life may depend on our response time, so we use our lights and siren to get through traffic and as a general warning to other vehicles to yield the right-of-way.

Unless qualified medical personnel at the scene advise us to proceed with caution, we must assume a life-threatening emergency and use all of our warning signals, even when the dispatch information indicates a relatively minor problem. All of our volunteers have experienced calls such as those in which a person feeling dizzy turned out to be in cardiac arrest or when a hip injury turned out to be massive head trauma.

On the other hand, there are situations in which use of our lights and siren can have an adverse effect on a patient. An emotionally disturbed patient may become more agitated. A heart attack patient may become more anxious. There can even be direct physiological effects. The rhythmic flashing of the strobe lights on the top of the ambulance can trigger a seizure in an epileptic patient.

Family members or friends frequently accompany our patients to the hospital. One non-patient can ride in the ambulance with us, although we usually request that he ride in the cab with the driver. That keeps civilians out of our way, particularly when the condition of the patient in the back is serious.

When approached by an ambulance, drivers of other cars do strange things. They may pull over to the right, as they are required to do by law. Sometimes, however, they pull to the left and sometimes they just come to a stop in the middle of the road, unsure of what to do. Occasionally, a driver on a cross street stops so suddenly that the car behind him cannot react quickly enough to avoid a fender bender. We've had to use our ambulance radio to report several of those.

Once he sees the ambulance pass, a driver will frequently pull his car in behind us, thinking that he will get through traffic more quickly that way. A car containing a family member, rushing to the hospital behind us, will occasionally get into an accident with such a driver.

Family members also tend to tailgate the rig. I've had to climb out of the back of the ambulance on a few occasions and talk to some upset family member or friend of our patient, warning them to back off.

Therefore, we strongly advise friends or family, driving to the hospital with our patient, not to follow the rig.

FIVE

THE SOUND OF the Hurst Tool, otherwise known as the jaws of life, is unmistakable. The gasoline-powered compressor engine of the tool pulses and drones so that, as Ed and I got out of his car and ran toward the crumpled cars 20 feet down the parkway, we knew that at least one victim was trapped in the wreckage.

The pagers had gone off six minutes earlier, at 2:53 A.M. "Fairfax police to all home pagers, portables, and monitors. Two EMTs and an attendant are needed for a second rig at the scene of a personal injury auto accident just north of the Route 42 entrance to the northbound parkway. All available units, please call in. Fairfax Police clear."

I hadn't been awakened by the insistent beeping of my pager. Rather, I had been roused moments before by the sound of sirens. Since I've become a member of a volunteer ambulance corps, sirens have assumed a special meaning. I can differentiate between the wail of a police siren, the whine of the fire engines, and the yelp of the ambulance. Within the last five minutes, I had heard all three and that meant trouble.

"Wanna go?" Ed mumbled, not quite awake.

"Sure." I grabbed the phone, pressed the preprogrammed button to call the police. As the electronic beeps told me the phone was dialing, I propped the receiver against my ear and began pulling on my clothes.

"Fairfax Police, dispatcher Thomas."

"It's Joan Lloyd. Ed and I will respond directly to the scene." Because headquarters is north of my condo and Route 42 is south, that made sense.

"Thanks, Joan," the dispatcher said. "I have another EMT getting the rig." As it was late spring, during an unusual spell of hot weather, dressing took only moments. Less than two minutes after the pagers sounded, Ed and I were speeding toward the scene.

As Ed drove and I plugged the connector for Ed's green light into the cigarette lighter, we heard, "Be advised 45–02 is responding to the parkway at Route 42." I recognized Marge Talbot's voice. Good. En route already. That meant that the second rig should arrive only moments after we did.

I opened Ed's glove compartment and put on a pair of latex gloves. Then I put a pair in Ed's lap for him to put on as soon as he stopped the car.

Adrenaline pumping, Ed and I arrived at the scene of the accident. Although the pulse of the Hurst tool made talking difficult, Steve Nesbitt, the crew chief of the duty rig, filled us in.

"It was a head-on," he told us. It failed to register until later that a head-on on that stretch of the parkway, where the three lanes in each direction are separated by a 40-foot grassy median, was very unusual. "Victims in both cars are pinned, so the firemen decided to start with that one." Steve pointed to what was left of a two-door tan something-or-other. Because the front end was completely crushed and the rest was surrounded by a sea of black and yellow fire department turnout coats, it was impossible to tell exactly what kind of vehicle it had been before the accident.

"There's a man pinned in the driver's seat. His vitals stink, but he's conscious. He has at least one, possibly two broken legs. He's also got some facial lacerations. It'll be awhile before they can get him out. Tom and Heather are with him." Tom and Heather Franks were a young married couple who often rode midnights together. He was a strong

EMT and, although she was new to the corps, she was learning fast.

"Where do you want us?" Ed asked.

"Ed, you work with Bob and Nick in that car," Steve said, motioning toward the second vehicle that had once been a hatchback but now was merely a pile of crumpled dark-blue metal. A fireman was working on the passenger side door. "They are trying to gain access with the pry bar until the Hurst Tool is available." I assumed that Bob Fiorella and Nick Abrams were on the far side of the car working on the driver who was pinned inside. Ed sprinted off toward the pile of equipment on the ground next to the hatchback. I saw the collar bag, a green KED, a longboard, and the large crash bag.

I heard the siren of the second rig. "Joan," Steve said to me, "let's get extrication equipment from the second rig. Then you can work with Heather and Tom in that other car. We'll decide where Marge is needed as we go along. I'll maintain scene control."

I waited until 45–02 came to a stop, then helped Steve remove the stretcher. I pulled open the rear compartment door, grabbed the long backboard we would need, and loaded it onto the stretcher. Marge had already gotten another collar bag and KED. I took out the crash bag and added it to the pile on the stretcher, then dropped on a bag of extra straps as well.

Marge and I dragged the loaded stretcher next to what was left of the tan auto and asked Tom Franks for a quick rundown. "I thought the patient had possible bilateral femur fractures," he said, "but on palpation it seems to be only one knee that's injured. He also has extensive facial trauma with a lot of blood and serious damage to his left eye."

"How are his vitals?" I asked.

"Not too good. Respiration's rapid and shallow and his pulse rate is increasing. He's conscious and alert, though."

Suddenly, the pulsing of the Hurst Tool ceased and the firefighters set the heavy machine down. Three firemen pulled at the driver's side door until it was flush against the front fender, allowing us access to our patient.

"Where do you want me?" I asked Tom.

"Heather's the littlest of us," Tom said of his wife, "so she's probably best in the backseat." Someone had already used the window punch to remove all the car's windows so Tom helped Heather into the backseat, through the back window.

"How do you want to take him out?" Marge asked.

"Let's not waste time with a full immobilization. Let's take care of his face, support his knee, and get him out."

Marge and I agreed. I went around to the passenger side of the car and climbed in through the window. Heather had stabilized the patient's head, but she was too new to realize the importance of conversation.

"Try to calm down," I said to the patient as I took the gauze pads and roller bandage that Marge handed me. "We're taking good care of you. What's your name?"

"José," he mumbled.

"Hello, José, my name is Joan."

I heard Tom yell for Marge to hand him a "short" cervical collar and the EMT shears, so I began to explain what was happening. "That's Heather behind you with her hands on your head. She's young and gorgeous, but that guy cutting your shirt is her husband, so don't get fresh."

"Hi, José," Heather said.

"Hello," José said. "My legs hurt and my head. And how's my car? Is it totaled?"

The man's face was covered with blood, as was the front of his T-shirt. There was still blood flowing down his right cheek. Mindful as I am of anyone's blood, I glanced down at my gloved hands. As I had suspected, the gloves were shredded from the broken metal and glass pieces. "Marge," I yelled out the window. "Hand me another pair of gloves." I dusted my hands on the seat of my pants to remove any bits of glass, then pulled new gloves on over the ones I was already wearing.

"I'm going to check your face," I said to José, "and then I'll put on some bandages to control the bleeding and protect your eyes." I pressed on his forehead, cheekbones, and jaw. "Anything that I'm doing hurt?" I asked.

"How's my car? Did they have to cut my car up?"

"Let's get you taken care of," Heather said, "then we can worry about your car."

Blood was still flowing from several deep facial lacerations, and his face was so covered that I couldn't tell yet about the condition of his eyes. One or both eyes could have been seriously damaged.

"Does your face hurt where I pressed it?" I asked again.

"No," José said as I covered two severe cuts and both eyes with four-by-fours, "but how's my car?"

I was worried about his sight, and he was worried about his car. It always amazes me how people react to stressful situations.

As I wound the Kling bandages around José's head, Tom cut off the remainder of his T-shirt and checked his chest. "Anything hurt in here?" Tom asked.

"No, man," José said. "But my head and my legs hurt so bad."

As Tom and I arranged the cervical collar around José's neck, I heard the sound of the Hurst Tool begin again, this time on the other car. I briefly wondered what Ed was doing, but I was too involved with José to think about it for long.

"That thing on my neck's cold, man," José said.

"I know the plastic's cold," I said. "Just be patient for a little longer."

Marge handed Tom a non-rebreather face mask, already attached to an oxygen cylinder, and Tom placed it over José's face. "That's just some oxygen," Tom reassured José. "Try to breathe easily."

"You've got some facial cuts, so we're bandaging both your eyes just to be on the safe side." I looked at the front windshield and saw the spiderweb crack where my patient's face had hit it.

"What about my eyes?" José asked the question in an almost matter-of-fact manner. He had been more excited about his car. The question of his sight seemed almost academic to him.

I considered my answer carefully. I had learned very early in my career as an EMT never to lie to a patient, so I merely said, "Eyes are very well protected and usually survive this kind of accident well, but we need to protect them and keep them from moving. Tell me what happened."

"The car came from nowhere," José said.

"Which way were you driving?" I asked, adding another layer of bandages to José's face.

"South."

I wondered whether he realized that we were now on the northbound side. I saw Tom put the earpieces of a stethoscope in his ears and nod to me. Because we take many calls together, Tom and I could often communicate without words.

"José, I need you to take a deep breath. Can you do that?" I saw him start to nod, so I quickly added, "Don't nod, just breathe."

He took a deep breath and Tom listened to the air move through his lungs. "Answer my questions with your mouth and hold your head still. Any pain when you breathe?" I asked.

"No, it's okay."

"Good. Tell me exactly what hurts."

"My face and my left knee."

I kept asking questions, partly to assess the extent of his injuries, partly to continually assess his level of consciousness, and partly just to keep him talking. I reached down and gently touched José's knee. His pant leg was sticky with blood and he screamed when I touched him. "Do you have pain anywhere else?"

"No. I don't think so. How's my car?"

I ignored his question. "I need a scissors to get his jeans out of the way so I can check his knee."

Tom handed me the shears he had been using, and I quickly cut away José's pant leg and examined his knee.

"Some deep lacerations and abrasions on the knee and deformity in the upper tib-fib."

I reached down toward José's feet. "Can you feel me touching your toes?"

"Yeah."

"Wiggle the toes of your left foot for me." I felt his toes move through his sneakers. "Now the right, José." Again his toes moved correctly. I found pedal pulses in each foot. Good. No circulatory or neurological impairment.

"Do you think my knee's broken?"

"We can't tell yet. We'll get you to the hospital where they'll be able to take X-rays to find out and fix it if it is broken."

"Oh, my poor car."

"Let's move," I heard Tom say.

"Now, we're going to move you out of here," I explained. "It's going to hurt when we move you, but we've no choice."

"Okay. Shit, my face and my knee hurt." He hesitated. "Sorry about the language, lady."

"No problem. I've heard much worse. You've got to hold very still while we work, and don't try to help us. And if you're good, I'll teach you the most important part of being an EMT. If you can learn this, you'll know about fifty percent of what we do."

Carefully, we put one end of the longboard onto the edge of the seat and had two firemen support the other end. We swiveled José's body an eighth of a turn, and I began to move his legs into a better position. As I worked, I talked loudly, trying to take José's mind off the pain we were causing. "There are two main points to learn if you're going to understand EMTing. First, if it ain't broke, don't fix it. Second, and this one's particularly for you, if it hurts when you do this, don't do this. Got that?"

"You're one crazy broad," José said, a slight smile in his voice.

"I know that." I had his right leg on the seat and reached around trying to support his broken left one. "Okay, guys," I said, "let's do it."

José screamed as Tom and Marge rotated his body until his back was facing the nonexistent driver's side door.

"Okay, babe," I said to him, "we're almost ready to get you out of here. I'll warn you in advance that it will hurt that knee like hell, but we're doing our best."

Marge took over head stabilization from Heather, and Heather climbed back out the rear window. While Marge held his head, Tom and Heather guided José's chest and shoulders until his upper body was lying on the longboard.

Now we had to slide José's body along the board and out of the car. Tom and Heather took the young man's shoulders, and I supported his legs, paying special attention to his injured knee. When we were all in position, Marge, still holding head stabilization, said, "On my count. One, two, three!"

"Mother of God!" José screamed as his body started to move.

"There's no easy way, folks," Tom said as everyone hesitated. "Let's just do it."

"Hang on," I said to José. "This will suck the big one for a few moments, then it will be better."

"It will what . . . ?" José said as the four of us adjusted our position to get the best grip.

"You heard me, it will suck the big one."

Despite his pain, José chuckled. "You're quite something, lady," he said.

"On my count," Marge said again. "One, two, three!"

Somehow, we managed to get José out of the car and onto the longboard. Swiftly, we fully immobilized his knee and leg and strapped down his body. We added more gauze to one area where the blood had soaked through the existing dressing and immobilized his head to the board. Moments later we lifted the stretcher, with José on it, into the rig. Marge switched the oxygen to the main on-board tank, then went around to the driver's seat.

"Joan," José called, pulling one arm loose from the straps and waving it blindly, "are you here with me?"

"Right here," I answered climbing into the back of the ambulance. "And I'm going to the hospital with you, too. You're not getting rid of me that easy. I have a few more things to teach you about being an EMT."

José clutched my hand and held it tightly. "Thanks."

Tom took a quick set of vitals. "BP ninety-six over seventy-four. Pulse ninety-four, respirations twenty-four. He seems to be stabilizing."

"That's good, José," I said. "Just try to relax. We're on our way to the St. Luke's Trauma Center. It's a terrific facility, and they'll be able to fix you up."

We were ready to roll with Marge driving, Tom, Heather, and me in the back. As we pulled away, the sound of the jaws continued. I looked over at the dark-blue hatchback and saw that the woman was still trapped.

As Joan gathered equipment to attend to her patient, I ran over to Bob and Nick next to the dark-blue hatchback. The car had obviously rolled once, pressing the roof about one foot into the headspace of the passenger compartment, now flattened to about half its size. Neither of the doors would open and the metal was so contorted that we couldn't gain full access to the patient through any of the windows.

"Shit, what a mess," I said. "What can I do?"

"Glad you're here, Ed," Nick said. "The firefighters pried us some space through the driver-side window opening and Bob's tending to the woman through there, but we have to get someone into the car. Ideas?"

"How about the hatch?" I said. I grabbed a fireman. "Have you got a window punch?"

The fireman nodded. "What do you want done?"

"The hatch," I said. "We need you to pop the window in the hatch."

"Will do." We accompanied the fireman around to the back of the car and watched as he stretched several lengths of duct tape across the window to keep shards of glass from flying. He then pressed the punch to the lower right-hand corner several times. The third press resulted in the satisfying pop of the shattering safety glass. The fireman used his hands, protected by heavy work gloves to pull the sheet of plastic, glass, and tape clear of the frame.

"I'll go," I said. Because I was the smallest EMT around, I put on one of our big yellow crash helmets, crouched down, and carefully climbed through the new opening and into the backseat. My first job was to hold head stabilization on the woman, still trapped in the driver's seat. In addition, she would need a lot of psychological first aid while the firefighters cut the car with the jaws and did the necessary forceful extrication.

As I climbed, trying to move the car as little as possible, I said to the woman, "My name's Ed. What's yours?"

"Louise."

"Okay, Louise, tell me where it hurts." I scrunched down in the backseat and reached around the headrest to support the woman's head.

"My feet are tangled around the pedals, and I think my left leg or hip is broken. My left arm and shoulder hurt like crazy."

"Are you having any trouble breathing?"

"No. Not really."

"Any pain in your head, neck, or back?"

"No. Just my shoulder and arm and my hip."

"Did you black out during the accident?"

"I don't think so. But I'm pretty scrambled and I don't remember exactly how the accident happened."

"That's perfectly normal. You've had a tough few minutes." I saw that the firefighters had freed the man Joan was working on and were now setting the Hurst Tool up next to the car I was in. "Things are going to get a bit noisy now while those guys cut away enough of the car so we can get you out."

I could feel the woman shudder beneath my hands. "It's all right, Louise. I'll be right here with you. Now, we need one more thing." I signaled to Bob, who carefully draped a heavy canvas blanket over both of us.

"What's that for?" the terrified woman screamed.

"That's just to protect us from any glass or metal that might fall on us. We'll be fine." I nodded to the turnout-geared firefighters and they started up the compressor.

"Just please get me out," she cried. "It hurts so much and I'm scared."

"We are going to get you out as quickly as possible," I told her as the weight of the cover pressed my heavy helmet onto my forehead. "First the firemen have to get the door off the car. It's going to be loud and you may feel the car move, but don't be scared. We're safe under this tarp."

What she didn't realize was that I was trying to ease my own fears as well as hers. I knew that her left leg and hip were almost touching the door. I had no idea how the hell they were going to open up the car without causing her more pain.

I am always frightened when I am inside a car while it is being pried apart by a Hurst Tool. Under the tarp that protects you from flying glass and debris you can't see what is going on. You hear the pulsing drone of the compressor and the terrifying noises of the steel vehicle being torn apart. You have to trust that the firefighters know what they are doing and that they will not cause a suddenly released piece of metal to slice into your body or that of your patient. I never really trust them completely, but there's nothing I can do until they complete their job except try to encourage myself and my patient.

The churning sound of the air compressor started, and we could hear metal creaking and groaning. I could imagine the giant reverse scissorlike jaws prying an opening between the door and its frame, trying to get to the door-locking mechanism. With luck, the door lock would quickly pop open.

"What were you doing out this late at night?" I asked, keeping my voice light.

"I work the six P.M. to two A.M. shift at an answering service. God, I hate it under here."

"I know. What kind of answering service?"

"Like for doctors. My husband works days, and he comes home and takes care of the kids. That noise is so loud I can't hear myself think."

I felt myself begin to sweat, as much from fear as from the hot, stagnant air under the tarp. We could not see what was happening, but we could hear the sounds of metal straining and snapping and the drone of the compressor.

"How old are your children?" I asked, trying to keep my voice from trembling.

"They're six and four." Suddenly Louise began to shriek. "Oh, God, they're cutting my hip. They're cutting my hip." She frantically tried to move her body away from the jaws. I was afraid that she would aggravate her injuries.

"Stop," I yelled to the firefighters, but they couldn't hear me over the noise. I partially raised the tarp and leaned over until I could see her hip. "They've made an opening around the door," I told her, "and what you feel is just the compressor hose sticking through that opening. It's not anything that can hurt you."

"Are you sure?"

I slid my right hand across the woman's forehead to support her head. Then I slipped my left hand down the side of the seat and placed my hand on her hip. "Can you feel my hand on your side?" I asked.

"Yes," she answered, tears rolling down her face.

"I am going to keep my hand there," I told her. "They can't cut your hip without cutting my hand and you can believe that I wouldn't let them cut my hand. You have to trust me."

"Thank you," she whispered, beginning to relax while her car was cut and pried from around us.

The noise stopped so abruptly that the sudden silence was deafening. I could hear the screech of protesting metal, and then it was over. Bob pulled the heavy canvas off of our heads, and Louise and I looked around. The driver's side door was gone and the roof of the car had been peeled back.

"Are they done?" Louise asked.

I took a deep breath. "I sincerely hope so." I looked at Bob, and he nodded.

"You're sweating and shaking," Louise said. "Were you scared? You didn't seem to be."

"Well, if you want me to be totally honest, I hated it under there worse than almost anything."

"But you seemed so calm."

I chuckled. "Shows how much you know. Now, let's get you out of here."

Bob examined her. "Ow," she screamed again as he touched her upper left leg, then she screamed as he touched her left arm and shoulder.

"Oh, God, it hurts so much."

Bob checked her feet and hands. "Pulses and neuros intact," he said.

"What does that mean?" Louise asked me.

"It means that you seem to be in one piece." I kept head stabilization and continued talking to Louise while the others worked.

"Ed, I think we should fully immobilize her before we get her out. Agree?"

"I do."

Bob took a cervical collar from the collar bag and quickly fastened it around Louise's neck. Then he pulled the green KED from its sleeve and slipped it between Louise's back and the seat. He pulled the side pieces under her arms and across her chest. With Bob's support, I adjusted my grip so I held stabilization with my hands around the extrication device's headpieces. Thanks to the removal of the roof, Nick was able to climb over the passenger-side door and settle himself in the passenger seat.

With Nick's help, Bob straightened the jacket and fastened two of the KED's three sets of body straps. "Middle," he said, coordinating his hand with Bob's, "and bottom." I heard two snaps as the male and female ends of the straps locked. "Now the legs," Bob said. Working together, Bob and Nick worked the leg straps up between Louise's thighs and fastened them to the side connectors.

"We're almost done now," I said to my patient. "Only a few more straps to go. There's a way we remember what order they should be attached, you know. We use the phrase 'Marlon Brando lost his toupee.' " Bob and Nick now used Kling bandages to affix Louise's head to the KED, and I continued talking to the frightened woman. "That stands for middle, bottom, legs, head, and, finally, top." Nick pulled the top body strap across the woman's chest.

"I know it's not comfortable," I continued, "but it's not designed for comfort. The jacket is to keep you from moving until the hospital can be sure you've got no spinal injuries. It's just a precaution, but an important one."

"I don't have any pain in my neck or back, you know."

"I know, but we have to do this to keep you safe."

"Okay, if you think it's important."

It had taken only five minutes to immobilize Louise's body, and finally we could get her out of the vehicle onto a long spine board. As we loaded her into the ambulance, I thought about Joan, probably almost at the hospital by now.

St. Luke's is geared for trauma. When Heather, Tom, Marge, and I arrived with José, in spite of the fact that it was almost 4 A.M., a full trauma team was ready for him. A technician drew blood while a nurse started an IV. A second nurse cut the bandages from José's eyes while Dr. Englander, a doctor who specialized in the treatment of trauma patients, looked over her shoulder. "Call X-ray," he ordered. "I'll need pictures of his head and neck and one of his knee."

As we helped the staff remove the tape and straps from the longboard, I heard the nurse say, "The facial damage is not as extensive as it might be."

I watched Dr. Englander palpate and probe. "Severe lacerations and a possible orbital fracture, but the globe of the eye appears intact." That was excellent. Stitches and plastic surgery would be required, but his vision could probably be saved.

"That's good news, José," I said as I squeezed his hand one last time. "Listen. I'm going to leave you now, but these folks here will take the best care of you."

"Thanks, again, lady," José said.

As we cleaned up and remade the stretcher with clean linen, we waited for Ed and the crew with the second patient. A few moments later, I heard Bob Fiorella's voice over the hospital radio. "St. Luke's, this is Fairfax 45–02."

"Go ahead, 45–02."

"We are en route to your location with a twenty-eight-year-old female, the victim of a head-on motor vehicle accident. She is complaining of pain in her left hip, shoulder, and arm. We have the arm and shoulder splinted, and she is on a longboard with O_2 at twelve liters via non-rebreather face mask. Her vitals are: pulse eighty and regular, respirations twenty-four and shallow, and her BP is one hundred and ten over eighty. The patient is conscious and alert. Our ETA is about five minutes."

"10–4, 45–02. We'll be expecting you. St. Luke's clear."

"How the hell did those two survive?" Steve asked from behind me. "One look at those cars and I expected dual fatalities."

Less than five minutes later, Ed and the other members of the crew wheeled the woman into an exam room where the trauma team went to work. Dr. Englander ordered X-rays of her leg, arm, and shoulder, and a nurse started an IV and drew blood for type and cross-matching in case of internal injuries.

While Bob and Marge filled out PCRs, the rest of us quickly went through the two rigs, both now filled with half-used trauma bags, open bandages, gauze, tape, oxygen masks, and bottles. We wanted to return order to at least one of the rigs, so we transferred enough equipment to get 45–01 back into service. 45–02 would need replacement supplies when it returned to headquarters. By the time both rigs left the hospital parking area, the ER staff had started IVs on the second patient and were preparing both patients for X-ray. Both Louise and José would be all right.

* * *

Twenty minutes later, as the first light appeared in the eastern sky, Ed and I arrived back at the accident scene in 45–01 so we could pick up his car. It was light enough now to see the skid marks. It seemed that José had fallen asleep and crossed the median. At that hour of the morning, with traffic usually very light, it was amazing that he had hit another car and not just driven into the woods. That was Louise's bad luck. Because Steve and Marge had volunteered to clean up, we headed home.

As we arrived back at my condo, dawn had broken and the birds had awakened. "Listen," Ed said. "The bird music is so loud and the sky is fantastic."

"Life goes on," I mumbled as I looked at the pink and gray sunrise. "Life goes on."

I got a few hours of sleep after that call, and I kept dreaming that I was at the scene of a serious accident and I was doing my work naked. I don't know whether the dream reflected my feeling that we are all so vulnerable to the acts of others, like the woman driving north, unaware of someone falling asleep behind the wheel of a southbound vehicle, or that we EMTs are naked and exposed when we care for our patients. We work without a hospital support staff of nurses and technicians, without sophisticated equipment like X-rays and IVs, often without all the hands and help we would like. But we do it and at Fairfax VAC, we do it well.

A few days later, we read in the paper that both patients were treated, held through the next night, then released from the hospital.

○ ○ ○

THERE WAS NO crew on duty that morning, so I was closely monitoring my portable radio. I knew that at the other end of town Joan was doing the same. Either or both of us would respond if a call came in.

Suddenly the radio emitted a series of tones, followed by the voice of the police dispatcher.

"Fairfax police to all Fairfax Ambulance Corps monitoring units. An ambulance is needed at 1254 Franklin for an unknown medical emergency. Please call in."

"Fairfax Police, Dispatcher Thomas speaking."

"Hi, Mark," I responded. "Has anyone called in?"

"Just Joan," he replied. "She's going to pick up the rig."

"Okay. Tell her I'll meet her at the scene. And set off the pagers again for at least one more crew member."

The radio came alive as I headed toward my car. "Fairfax Police to 45–24. 45–22 will meet you at the scene."

As I got into my car and placed the green light on the roof, the pager tones sounded again.

"Fairfax Police to all Fairfax Ambulance personnel. One more crew member is still needed for an unknown emergency at 1254 Franklin. Please call in."

As I drove down my quiet residential street, I plugged my green emergency light into the cigarette lighter. At first I didn't notice the tendril of blue smoke that began to drift from under the dashboard.

Soon, however, I noticed the awful smell. I sniffed the air, looked down, and saw that smoke was pouring into the car. By the time I could bring the car to a stop, it was already filled with heavy acrid smoke. I threw open the door, instinctively grabbed my radio and stumbled out of the car, choking and gasping for breath. I had taken only one or two breaths of the smoke, but I felt as if my lungs had been seared. I had treated firefighters for smoke inhalation, but I had never experienced it myself.

I stood outside my car for a few unbelieving seconds, watching the smoke pour out of the car and trying to breathe. Keying the microphone, I croaked into the radio. "45–22 to Fairfax Police." As soon as the words were out of my mouth, I started to cough.

"Fairfax Police on. Go ahead 45–22."

I saw a tiny flame from below the car heater controls. "Can't respond to call," I said through my coughs. "Car's on fire. Get fire department to Orchard and Sycamore."

As I struggled to breathe, my stomach began to heave. I keyed the mike again. "Get an ambulance here, too."

I sat on the curb, gasping for breath, watching my car burn and listening for the wailing sounds of emergency vehicles that would be coming for me this time.

I swung into the Ambulance Corps parking lot, turned off my green light, leapt from my car, and sprinted toward the ambulance. Steve Nesbitt was behind the wheel and was waiting for me. "Jump in, Joan. Ed's meeting us at the scene."

As I slid into the passenger side, Steve pulled the microphone from the control panel.

"45–01 to all units. Be advised, 45–01 is responding to an unknown medical emergency at 1254 Franklin Street."

"Unknown medical emergency." That could be anything from an infected hangnail to a massive heart attack. I hate calls that come in as "unknown medical." They give me no chance to prepare for the logistical or psychological requirements of the call. Would they need the defibrillator or just the crash bag? Would it be a hysterical parent, terrified by an infant's fever-caused convulsions, or would we have to "work a code"—attempt to resuscitate someone in cardiac arrest.

We could hear bursts of heavy static from the radio, and we heard the police respond to something Ed said.

Suddenly, two familiar musical tones blared from the radio. I looked at Steve. "Another call?"

"Fairfax Police to all pagers and monitors. A second ambulance is needed for smoke inhalation at a car fire at the intersection of Orchard and Sycamore. Also, one more member is needed to respond to the call at 1254 Franklin. All available units please call in."

"Orchard and Sycamore is right near Ed's house," I said, making some quick assumptions. "He must have passed the fire and stopped to help."

When we arrived at the house on Franklin, we parked the ambulance behind the Fairfax Police patrol car, got the crash bag, and went up the narrow walkway to the front door. We were met at the door by a weeping woman.

"My father stopped breathing," she cried. "Please hurry."

Dave Hancock arrived, and the three of us worked the code. After three shocks from the defibrillator, the seventy-four-year-old man had converted from ventricular fibrillation, a disorganized heart rhythm incapable of supporting life, to asystole, flat line, no electrical heart activity. "The machine won't shock anymore," I said. "Let's transport."

We commandeered Chuck Harding, a Fairfax policeman, to drive and sped to the hospital doing CPR in the back of the rig.

We arrived at the ER and backed the ambulance in beside the other Fairfax rig. We quickly wheeled our patient into cubicle 4, the one devoted to cardiac care. As I bent down to unfasten the stretcher straps, I felt something snap in my back. I tried to straighten up, but couldn't. I'd had problems with my back before, and I recognized the sensations. I knew the pain would come soon, but at that moment it wasn't too bad. I just couldn't straighten up, couldn't unfasten the strap, couldn't move at all.

"What's the matter, Joan?" Steve asked.

"I think my back went out," I said. "I can't move."

I wonder where Ed is, I thought. He should be here with the smoke inhalation patient. At least that's lucky. He can drive me home and give me some TLC.

With some heat and massage, I knew I'd be all right in a week or so. Back problems are almost endemic among EMTs. We work in cramped quarters, move heavy patients, and frequently abuse our bodies by lifting with our backs, not our legs as we know we should.

"Give me a hand," I said to Stephanie DiMartino. I assumed she had been with Ed and the smoke inhalation patient.

While Steve, Dave, and the ER staff worked on our cardiac arrest patient, Stephanie helped me onto a gurney in cubicle 2, so I could get my back flat for a few moments and catch my breath. I was beginning to hurt a lot. "Where's Ed?" I asked Stephanie. "And how's the smoke inhalation patient?" With a flourish, Stephanie pulled back the curtain between cubicles 1 and 2.

I gasped as I saw Ed, sitting up, with a non-rebreather oxygen mask covering his nose and mouth. His eyes were closed. "You're the smoke inhalation?" I said. I could see that he was struggling to breathe without coughing. "Are you okay?"

Ed opened his eyes and looked at me, flat on my back on the gurney. I answered his unspoken questions quickly so he wouldn't try to talk. "My back went out as we arrived here. Are you okay?"

Immediately he gave me the thumbs-up sign. "Talking's hard," he said. "You?"

"I'll be fine," I said. "My back's been this bad before. It'll just take time. I was hoping for some TLC."

"So was I."

We stared at each other for a few seconds, then, simultaneously burst out laughing. Ed's laughter was quickly interrupted by a gasping cough, and mine was cut short as I moved and the pain brought tears to my eyes.

In less than a week, each of us was fully recovered. Never before or since has anyone been hurt on a Fairfax ambulance call, and here we both were injured on the same call, five miles apart.

HOW I BECAME AN EMT

UNTIL 1985, WHEN Ed and I started dating, I had never paid much attention to our local ambulance corps. I had received their semiannual fund drive letters, and I regret to say that I had never contributed. I felt, as so many people do, that when I needed an ambulance I would dial 911 and an ambulance would magically appear in my driveway. I had no idea of how the system worked and how much goes into an ambulance response. By then, Ed had been a member for more than ten years.

One summer Tuesday morning, Ed asked me to go with him while he assisted an ambulance crew. "I saw Pam Kovacs and Jack McCaffrey at the corps yesterday afternoon. They're doing a transport this morning, and they can use a hand."

"They're what?" Ambulance jargon.

"Sorry. They're doing an ambulance transport. That's a noncritical request to drive a patient, usually someone who's bedridden, from one place to another. In this case, we're transporting an older man from his home to the hospital. He's a terminal cancer patient going in for chemotherapy."

"Okay, what do they need you for?" The idea of being part of an ambulance call scared me a little. It sounded so serious.

"They need lifting help. The man's wife says he weighs more than 200 pounds, and there are several stairs from the front door to the driveway. I won't take long. That okay with you?"

Of course it was. We got to the patient's house and, while I waited in the car, Ed disappeared inside. A few minutes later, he reappeared and walked over to me. "I could use a favor in a few minutes. Could you guide me down the stairs? I'll be walking backward and I won't be able to see my feet. If you would just stay behind me with your hand in the small of my back, counting steps out loud, it would be a big help."

I nodded, and Ed disappeared back inside the house. When he emerged, a woman in a white uniform shirt and navy-blue pants was wheeling a large man, bundled in a blanket, toward the top of a long flight of flagstone stairs. She was followed by Ed and another man, also in a white uniform shirt and navy pants, and a little white-haired woman. I got out of the car and walked up the stairs.

Ed quickly introduced me to the two crew members. "Pam and Jack are going to take the top handles," Ed explained, looking at me. "I'll take the bottom. You'll have to back me up."

Together the three EMTs guided the chair to the top of the stairs, then Ed took the handles at either sides of the foot of the chair and lifted. As he walked backward down the stairs, I walked behind him. "Five more steps, four, three, two, last one. You're down."

Panting, the three corps members set the chair down at the foot of the stairs. "Thank you so much," the patient wheezed. The woman I assumed to be the man's wife locked the front door and hurried down the front stairs. "I want to thank all four of you," she said, assuming that I was a member of the crew, "for helping us this way. I didn't know what to do. You've been so great."

That was when the itch started for me. It was that thank-you. I loved it. I began to think about myself in an ambulance context. I had raised two children and was no stranger to minor illnesses and childhood injuries. My daughters had had their share of stitches, vomiting, bumps, and bruises, but neither of them had ever been seriously ill or injured. How would I respond? I had no idea whether I could do it. But I didn't know that I couldn't either.

I broached the subject to Ed and he was delighted. "I would enjoy it so much if you took an EMT course," he said. "We could share so much. We could ride together. As a matter of fact, I don't mean to push you, but there's a course starting next month at Fairfax Hospital. I teach some of the lab skills."

"Do you really think I could do it?"

"I have no doubt in the world. You'd be wonderful." Ed was certainly more sure than I was. And anyway, I could always drop out.

By the second week in September, I had joined FVAC as a probationary member and started my EMT course. It was taught by an EMT instructor named Connie, her chief lab instructor Mark, and a number of other lab instructors, one of whom was Ed.

We began with CPR, and I picked that skill up quickly. Doing mouth-to-mouth on Resusci-Annie (the CPR mannequin) wasn't my idea of great fun, but once I got used to her less than lifelike face, she wasn't so bad. I was surprised that I had so little trouble learning CPR skills on the baby manikin. I did well working on a doll, but I had no idea how I might react to working on a real child. I could only hope that I would do what had to be done, then fall apart later.

We studied the first few techniques, patient assessment, oxygen and airways, and bleeding control and practiced both on manikins and on one another. I learned so much new terminology that I was sure that whatever I pushed into the front of my brain was causing as much stuff to fall out the back.

"Boy," I told Ed one evening, "I was a schoolteacher for many years, but I haven't sat in this part of a classroom in more than twenty years."

Then came our first practical-skills test. First, I walked into a room and found Resusci-Annie lying in the middle of the floor. The lab instructor/proctor told me that she had stopped breathing so, without too much hesitation, I went through the ABCs of CPR and started rescue breathing. When I was told that she now had no heartbeat, I combined my breaths with reasonably good chest compressions.

So far, so good.

"Joan," Connie said when I returned to the main classroom, "room three next."

I walked into room three and saw Ed sitting at the desk. He pointed to a body lying on the floor. "You've been called to the scene of an unknown medical emergency. You'll need to do a patient survey and tell me what you find," Ed said.

I froze. There was a real person lying on the floor, seemingly unconscious. Somewhere in my brain I knew that it was a member of the ambulance corps's youth group, pretending to be a patient, but that wasn't enough.

"Just do your survey," Ed said softly.

I couldn't move. "Joan?" Ed said again.

I turned and ran. I ended up in the bathroom, sitting on the white tile floor, sobbing. I couldn't do it. Not ever. I just couldn't.

I had been sitting there for about five minutes when Connie walked in. "It's all right," she said soothingly. "It happens more often than you can imagine."

"You mean other people have panicked like I did?"

"Lots. But they usually go back and try again. Are you riding with FVAC yet?"

"I have ridden about four shifts, but I haven't gotten any calls," I said, my lower lip still quivering.

"It takes time to get used to seeing someone like that," she said. "You will get used to it." She knew that Ed and I were dating. "Is it Ed? I can get someone else to grade you."

"It's not really Ed," I admitted. "I just had no idea what to do."

"Talk me through the survey right here," Connie said.

"Well, first you hold head stabilization and . . ." After about ten minutes, we left the bathroom together. "Ready?" she asked.

"I guess." I reentered room three and, without too much fumbling, surveyed my "patient," found and bandaged a "seriously bleeding wound" in his arm. I had to smile when I found the supposed injury, because on a piece of tape stuck to my patient's perfectly normal forearm, was a sign in large, red letters that said, "Seriously Bleeding Wound."

When I returned to our main classroom, Connie and I grinned at each other. "So you made it," she said.

"I did, I did." I pulled out my wallet, withdrew a $20 bill and walked over to the coffee kitty, an empty instant coffee bottle. "Let's see, at a dollar a session, this ought to get me through most of the rest of the class." I dropped the bill into the jar. "Now I'm committed to staying."

In the years since that first class, I've become a state-certified instructor coordinator, and I have taught several EMT courses myself. Somewhere, usually just before the first practical skills exam, I tell my class the story of me and Connie and my first skills exam and warn them about seeing "real patients." Maybe that's part of the reason that I've never had to rescue a student from the bathroom.

The first time I drove the ambulance in an emergency situation I was still a probationary member, still taking my EMT course with Connie. I had taken FVAC's driver-training course and had driven back to headquarters from the hospital, but I had never driven code 3.

Ed and I were on duty together when we received a call for a patient at a local doctor's office who needed to go to the hospital. We paged out for additional manpower, but, as we drove to the scene we realized that there was no one else available. A simple transport wouldn't be a problem. I would drive and Ed would tend to the patient.

As Ed drove to the scene, he used the lights and the siren to move traffic out of our way and get us to the scene quickly. I had been shown the complicated panel switches that controlled the wigwag, the grill lights, the alley lights, the bar flashers, and the dials that control the three sirens and the air horn. In my previous driving experiences, however, I had never had to use any of them. To refresh my memory, I watched which buttons Ed pushed and which knobs he turned just in case I needed to drive code 3. The siren controls didn't look too difficult and I wouldn't speed, just drive efficiently. Anyway, emergency driving probably wouldn't be needed. This was probably just a transport.

We picked up the patient, a man with severe abdominal pain, and loaded him into the ambulance. He was in agony, vomiting, and moaning. Ed checked his vital signs and settled into the back. "Move it, Joan," he said. "Fairfax Hospital, code 3."

"You got it," I said. I walked around and climbed into the ambulance driver's seat, recalling all the driving rules I had learned. But it wasn't the driving that presented the problem.

Ed is only five foot five and carries most of his height in his upper body. As I settled my five-foot-seven-inch body into the seat, I had a rude shock. The driver's seat was pushed all the way forward. This is an ambulance, I thought. It's a special kind of vehicle. I have no idea how to move the seat back to accommodate my long legs. I looked over the complicated control panels that operate the lights, sirens, and engine speed, I saw nothing labeled "seat control".

So I had no choice. I drove to the hospital with my back hunched forward and the steering wheel just clearing my thighs. I used the siren and the lights and enjoyed seeing traffic move out of my way. I made a full stop at each red light, then proceeded slowly through the intersections as I had been taught. I turned corners carefully, remembering that an ambulance is top-heavy and left-side unbalanced.

We arrived at the hospital, unloaded our patient, and transferred his care to the emergency room staff. While

Ed did the paperwork, I disposed of the used linen and replaced it with clean sheets, a clean cotton blanket, and a fresh pillowcase.

As we loaded the stretcher into the rig, Ed asked, "How did you like driving with lights and sirens? From the back it seemed to go well."

"It went fine, but I did have one problem," I laughed. "How do you move this damned seat?"

"Oh, God, I forgot that you need the seat all the way back." He climbed in and showed me the handle under the front seat. "It's just like a car. Nothing exotic."

"You're kidding. That simple? I feel like such a jerk. Oh, well. I managed. I did what I had to."

That's the way EMTs handle most situations. We do what we have to do.

Like my first experience with death. It was a few weeks after the seat incident. Ed and I were returning from a call. We had dropped off two other members to pick up their cars and were about to stop for gas.

"Fairfax Police to the ambulance corps. Dispatch an ambulance to the scene of an auto accident." The dispatcher gave the address, very near our location, and we called in that we were responding. The two members whom we had just dropped off radioed that they were responding to the scene also.

As we pulled up, even before the police, we saw a white Toyota, crushed against a tree in the middle of someone's front yard. We could see two people, a man and a woman, in the front seat both slumped over and not moving.

I grabbed the megaduffel (the large first-aid kit that we carry in the ambulance) and, following Ed, ran to the car. He quickly reached in through the driver's window and felt the driver's neck for a carotid pulse. At that moment, two other members arrived. "Take care of the passenger," Ed yelled to them. "Joan, let's get the driver out and onto the ground. There's no pulse."

As we pulled the man out, I got my first look at him. He was at least seventy, his face pasty white and slack.

Although he was a small man, I was shocked at how heavy he was.

As a police car pulled up, Ed yelled for the officer to call for more help and a second rig for the other victim.

We dragged the driver a short way across the grass and lay him out flat on the ground. Ed again checked for pulse and breathing and found none. *There's no bleeding,* I thought. *How can someone be dead with no bleeding?*

"You do ventilations, Joan, I'll do compressions. More help's on the way."

A few moments later a man came around the car and bent over our patient. "Stop CPR and move over, Ed," he said. "Let me examine him. The woman passenger's dead."

"Who's that?" I whispered, backing away from the patient.

"That's Dr. Margolis. He works in the ER at Fairfax General. He can pronounce."

Pronounce. That meant that this doctor could give us permission to stop CPR if he decided that the man was truly dead.

Dead. This man is dead. The woman, his wife, I presumed, is also dead. I looked into the man's face and tried to feel something. I waited for the pain of this man's death to begin. I felt nothing. What's wrong with me? I wondered. Have I no feelings? Why don't I feel something, some sadness?

The doctor stood up. "There's no use," he said. "He's dead. Probably ruptured an aorta on impact. He didn't feel a thing." He conferred with the police officers for a few moments, then said, "The police have canceled the second rig and you can go back to headquarters. They will take care of everything from here on."

As we drove back to headquarters, Ed said, "Lucky the doctor was around. Otherwise we would have had to do CPR all the way to the hospital. Then the doctor on duty in the emergency room would have pronounced."

We rode in silence. "What's wrong?" Ed asked. "Is this call getting to you?"

"No, it's not," I said, "and that's what's bothering me. I don't know what's wrong with me. I don't feel anything."

"You may feel it later, you may not. It's a funny thing about death the way we see it. We've never known these people alive, so seeing them dead isn't any kind of transition."

Ed sighed. "I remember my first code. On the way back from the hospital, the crew joked around. I found myself joining in, wondering, like you, whether I was ever going to feel anything. I've discovered that some you feel, others you don't, and you never know which ones will get to you. You just have to let yourself react in whatever way you need to. Don't judge."

To this day I try not to judge myself. Most of the time I succeed.

SIX

SOMETIMES, IT'S NOT the calls you remember, it's the people.

Ed and I were driving north to meet some friends for dinner. As we rounded a curve in the parkway, we saw a minivan off the side of the road, perpendicular to the roadway, its front end crumpled. One state police car had just arrived and the officer was setting out a flare pattern to warn other drivers of the accident.

Ed pulled our car off the roadside and approached the minivan's driver, a pretty blond who appeared to be in her late twenties or early thirties, and was still in the driver's seat. I went to the police officer and quickly ascertained that it had been a one-car accident and the driver was the only one injured. I returned to the van to see that Ed was tending to the patient.

"What do you need?" I asked Ed.

"Why don't you get into the backseat and hold head stabilization while I get the crash bag from my car."

I pulled on gloves and climbed into the backseat. "I'm going to hold your head," I said, "to keep you from moving." I put my hands on either side of her face and introduced myself. "My name's Joan," I said, "and that's Ed out there. We'll be taking good care of you."

"My name's MaryAnn," the woman said.

Ed came back and began a full body survey while I continued to support the woman's head. "What hurts?" he asked.

"My knees and my head and my hands. Are you with the ambulance?"

Ed quickly checked her injuries as I explained. "We were just driving by. We're with Fairfax Ambulance, but the local ambulance will be here soon. We'll stay with you until they arrive."

For ten minutes I chatted with the woman while Ed examined her and tended to a superficial but bloody head injury just above my fingers, some nasty gashes on her knees, and two very banged-up hands.

"Joan," she said softly, "you've been so nice. I have to tell you something."

"What?"

She took a deep breath. "I'm HIV-positive."

Both Ed and I have long since made our peace with the risk of both HIV and hepatitis. We've both taken hepatitis vaccine shots, and we've decided that universal precautions, gloves, appropriate hand washing, and the like are sufficient to make us comfortable in dealing with AIDS and HIV-positive patients. I could tell, however, that MaryAnn was uncomfortable.

"What would you like me to do about it?" I asked softly.

"I don't know," she whispered. "I just thought that, since I'm bleeding and you're holding my head and your hands are in my blood and all . . ."

"Thanks, MaryAnn," I said. "I'm wearing gloves and I'll take special care to wash my hands thoroughly after we're done here. You know, I decided long ago that either I'd have to become comfortable with dealing with patients like you or I wouldn't do this at all."

"I'm amazed that you said anything," Ed said to her.

"Me, too," MaryAnn said. "Before you got here, I had intended to say nothing. I figured you'd . . . well, you know . . . run away or something. But you two are so nice, I couldn't keep silent."

"Thanks for the good thoughts," Ed said. "Here in suburbia we don't think about AIDS much. There are probably people, particularly in the volunteer community, who haven't yet come to terms with the risks, but we're fine with it."

"You guys are probably in a lot of danger," MaryAnn said, her eyes glancing over the accident debris in the car. "All this broken glass and shredded metal. What if you cut yourself?"

"We take precautions," Ed continued. "We wear gloves and put on extras if they tear. We wear heavy work gloves when we don't have to examine a patient. We're careful. And you, of all people, should know that AIDS isn't spread that easily, especially by casual contact."

"I know," MaryAnn said. "But I worry."

"I'm glad you worry about us, but we're fine," I said. We heard the siren from the approaching ambulance. "May I tell the crew what you just told us?" I asked.

"I guess. Do you think they'll be okay with it?"

"I'm sure they will." I mentally crossed my fingers.

When the Prescott ambulance arrived, I told the crew about MaryAnn's condition, and they reacted as I had hoped they would. Without batting an eyelash, the crew chief said to MaryAnn, "That's okay. Don't worry. We'll take good care of you. Now, do you know what medications you're on?"

Most people are wonderful when you give them a chance. Without any undue fuss, the Prescott Ambulance crew fully immobilized MaryAnn and transferred her to their rig. They thanked us profusely for stopping and for our help, then drove away.

"I don't know whether I would have been so forthcoming in her situation," Ed admitted. "I guess I'd be afraid that the public hysteria would affect the quality of my care."

"I don't know either," I said. "But I would hope that everyone would be as unperturbed as that crew was." I can only hope.

○ ○ ○

SOME OF OUR patients react to their illnesses or injuries with anger, others with silence. Still others, the ones we particularly enjoy working with, react with humor and good feelings.

The accident occurred at three in the morning. Our patient's car was hit in the front of the passenger side by a driver who tried to pull out of a local watering hole and didn't negotiate the turn properly.

When Ed and I arrived, someone directed us to a heavyset woman lying on the grass. "I'm very scared," she said immediately. "I can't move my left leg or my right shoulder." While Ed took vitals, I examined her and determined that, among other injuries, the femur, or thighbone, of her left leg was broken. What complicated everything was the fact that her leg was twisted under her. This wasn't going to be easy.

"My name is Joan, and that's Ed. What's your name?"

"Eleanor. I'm really scared. Could someone stay with me?"

"Sure," Ed said. "I'll stay with you and tell you exactly what's happening."

"Thanks," she said. "Hold my hand?" Ed took her hand.

"Eleanor, we're going to have to straighten your leg and it's going to hurt like hell," I told her.

"I don't suppose I could vote against whatever you're going to do," she said, concealing her pain.

"I'm afraid we have no choice," I said.

With the help of two other EMTs, I prepared the Hare Traction Splint so that once we began we could immobilize her leg in as short a period of time as possible. While we worked, Ed stayed at Eleanor's head, holding her uninjured hand and explaining everything that was going to happen.

"I know you have to do whatever you must," she said. "Just do it and get it over with."

As we straightened her leg and pulled manual traction, the pain must have been almost unbearable, but Eleanor took it as best she could.

"Shit, shit, shit," she said, "that hurts so much. Fuck, fuck, fuck." She smiled. "You know, it helps to say all those words. I never curse, you know. Fuck, shit, fuck, shit." As quickly as we could, we applied an ankle hitch and positioned the Hare Traction Splint's metal frame under her leg.

Pulling manual traction on the injured limb should have relieved some of the pain, but Eleanor still seemed to be in agony. Tears ran down her face, but she continued to quip with us. "The bastard who hit me. Drunk as a fuckin' skunk. It's silly, but it feels so good to say exactly what I feel using whatever language I want."

I connected the hook on the frame of the splint to the hitch on Eleanor's ankle as Ed explained, "We're going to crank up the traction to your leg now. It should relieve most of the pain in your thigh."

"Crank away. Anything that works."

We cranked the winch mechanism and, as the machine stretched the thigh, I suddenly saw her heave a great sigh and give the thumbs-up sign. "Hey, that's great, guys. That feels much better." She panted and tried to catch her breath. "Now, you got one of those things for my shoulder?"

"Afraid not," Ed said, "but we're going to immobilize it real tight and get you to the hospital."

"Can you give me something for the pain? My leg feels better, but the rest of me hurts like a son of a bitch." She paused momentarily. "Boy, listen to me curse, will you."

"We don't give medications, but as soon as we get you to the hospital, they can give you something."

"Pink fizzy-wizzys, I hope. I'm trying to be brave, but I hurt so bad."

"I'll tell them to give you the best stuff," I said.

We immobilized Eleanor's shoulder as much as we could, then slid her onto a long backboard, transferred her to the stretcher, and lifted her into the ambulance.

"Sorry," I said. "I know this moving is hurting you, but it's almost done." We snapped the stretcher into the frame in the rig.

"Listen, you guys," she said, "you're doing just great." She was the patient, in terrible pain, yet she was reassuring us.

On the way to the hospital, she chatted and cracked jokes, screaming each time the ambulance hit a tiny bump. By the time we arrived at Fairfax Hospital, we felt like we had known one another for a long time.

We transferred Eleanor to the gurney at the hospital and I began to do my paperwork. As I worked, I overheard a conversation.

Kurt Bankcroft, an emergency room nurse, began his examination of Eleanor's thigh. "Don't mind me," he said. "I'm just using my hands to examine you."

"At another time, I might enjoy it," she said.

"Don't say that to me," Kurt said, a grin in his voice, "I'm the company pervert."

"That's okay," Eleanor said, her voice tight with pain, "I'm the company slut."

○ ○ ○

THERE WERE THREE of us riding that night, myself, my daughter Judy, who was a new EMT at the time, and another relatively new member. I had been having back spasms and at that moment I didn't realize how my inability to lift would figure into our late-night call.

The call for a man with abdominal pain came in at about 1:15 A.M., and the three of us met at headquarters. We drove to the patient's home and were greeted by the patient's wife. "Gerry is in the bedroom," she said. "Go up the stairs and turn left, go down the hall and he's around the corner to the right."

We could hear Gerry bellowing as we climbed the stairs and, when we arrived in the bedroom and saw him, we understood the enormity of our problem. He must have weighed at least 450 pounds and, dressed in huge sweatpants and an oversized sweatshirt, he looked like a caricature of a linebacker. As I rolled up his sleeve to take his blood pressure, I was amazed by the size of his forearms and biceps. I had to use an especially large BP cuff just to enclose his upper arm. And he was in acute pain. While we examined him, he alternately yelled at the top of his voice and apologized for himself.

"I've had this before," he moaned, "but it's never been this bad." He punctuated his speech with another yell. "It's pancreatitis. It's been getting worse for the last few hours, but I thought I could wait until morning. Sorry to bother you guys, but you gotta get me to the hospital."

Hospital, I thought, I have no idea how we're even going to get you down the stairs. The only way to move the man through the circuitous hallways and down the stairs was to use a stairchair, a narrow chair with wheels at the back. The hallway wouldn't be a problem, but the stairs were another matter entirely. The stairchair is usually carried by two people, one in front and one in back, although we could use three or four in a pinch if they could fit.

I looked at my two partners and the policeman and shrugged. We could call for extra manpower, but I didn't know of any four people capable of carrying Gerry down the stairs. I had visions of having to call the fire department and having them lift Gerry out the window using the bucket truck.

"We've got a problem, Gerry," I explained while I finished taking his vitals. "We've got to get you down stairs and . . ." I looked him over, "well, you're certainly no lightweight." He managed a small smile through his pain. "We need to use a stairchair to get you around the corners and down the stairs. Although we can wheel it part of the way, there are places where we have to lift you. I have to admit that I'm not sure how we're going to do that."

"That's no problem," Gerry said, panting with the exertion of talking. "Joe, Tiny," he yelled between spasms of pain, "get in here."

Two men, each almost as enormous as Gerry, appeared in the doorway. Tiny, I thought as I looked at the two tremendous men. The name's appropriate.

"Yeah, Gerry," one of them said, "how're ya doin'? Is there something you need?"

"These are my friends Joe and Tiny," Gerry said, introducing me to the two hulks. "We were having a little late-night card game when my pain began. They'll be glad to help." He turned to the two men, moaning as he moved. "They need to lift me to get me downstairs."

"Sure, we can lift you," Tiny said. I had a flash picture of an old Laurel and Hardy comedy in which they were trying to get a piano up the stairs in front of a mansion. Each time they got it to the top, it rolled back down. This was my patient and I had to make the decisions and, as big as these two were, I was still dubious. I looked from one to the other, then at Gerry. "Are you sure?"

"Don't worry, lady," the one introduced as Tiny said, "we're cabinetmakers and we lift heavy stuff every day. Just get out of the way and we'll take over."

When Judy and the policeman arrived upstairs with the stairchair, Tiny and Joe took over. They got Gerry wrapped in a blanket and into the chair. "Okay, ma'am," Tiny said. "Anything else before we move him?"

"Just try to be gentle. Any movement is causing him severe discomfort."

"Discomfort, my ass," Gerry moaned. "It hurts like a son of a bitch when I move."

"We'll be easy," Tiny said. With Joe at the back and Tiny holding the front of the chair, the two men lifted Gerry as though he weighed nothing and carried him through the hall and down the stairs. Together, they settled him on the stretcher. "Need help lifting him into the ambulance?" Tiny asked.

"I'm afraid so," I answered.

With no help from anyone else, the two men hoisted Gerry and the stretcher into the rig. "We'll be there later," Tiny said as Gerry's wife got into the passenger seat of the ambulance. "We'll just clean up here so your wife don't have to."

Gerry screamed in pain with every bump, but otherwise the trip to the hospital was uneventful. When I called in, I smiled as I asked for lifting help to get Gerry out of the rig. When we drove up, there was a muscular security guard waiting. He took one look at Gerry and called in reinforcements. It took seven of us to lift our patient down from the rig. I still have no idea how we would have managed if he and his wife had been alone when the attack began.

○ ○ ○

"FAIRFAX POLICE TO the ambulance corps. Dispatch an ambulance to a 10-2 at the intersection of Oak Hill and Floral Way."

"10–4," Stephanie DiMartino said into the mike. "45–01 en route to a PIAA at Oak Hill and Floral Way."

"En route at 14:13 hours."

We sped toward the scene, a bad intersection on the other side of town. We had been averaging one accident at that corner each week, and as we approached, we saw that the new traffic light was still shrouded in plastic. "Better late than never," I muttered.

As we pulled to a stop, Bob Fiorella and Nick Abrams jumped out of the back and Stephanie climbed out of her shotgun position. "Joan," Stephanie yelled at me as I pushed my foot down on the emergency brake, "we've got one in this car. See if anyone else is hurt."

I looked at the two vehicles, an older black Honda Prelude and a recent-model gray Dodge hatchback locked together in the center of the roadway. Although only a narrow, two-lane road, Oak Hill had recently become the main route from the center of town to the new Fairfax Central Mall. With the new Floral Court development now fully occupied, Floral Way was suddenly handling a large volume of traffic as well.

I saw Bob jog to the rig and open the extrication cabinet on the outside of the ambulance. The three of them were evidently going to do a full extrication on the driver of the Dodge. I went up to the crowd next to the Honda. "Anyone here injured?" I asked loudly.

"That crazy broad was the only one in that car," a nice-looking man in his early twenties said, "and I was the driver of this used-to-be Prelude." He pointed toward the crumpled car, then winced. "Fuckin' woman ran through the intersection. Slammed me broadside. I just got the car." He reached his hand up and rubbed the back of his neck.

Quickly, I walked up to him and said, "I want you to stand very still, sir, while I hold your head." I circled around behind him and put one hand flat on each side of his head. "Does your neck hurt?"

"Yeah, it does a little. But it can't be anything. I've been walking around. I'm just a little dizzy, that's all."

"What's your name?" I asked him.

"George. George Fowler."

"Okay, George, here's what's going to happen. I don't think there's anything wrong with your neck, but we need to take every precaution. We're going to put a collar around your neck to protect it, then lie you onto a board. We'll take you over to Fairfax General, and let them take some X-rays. Okay?"

"Sure, I guess."

"Fingers, toes, hands, feet, all feel fine? All wiggle?"

I could feel the man flex all his extremities. "Yeah, I feel fine."

"Did you hit your head or lose consciousness at any time?"

"I don't really know."

I looked at the windshield of George's car. There was a small, star-shaped crack on the driver's side. "Do you remember the accident? Do you recall hitting your head?"

"Actually, I don't remember much about what happened. I just remember that asshole broad speeding toward me. She must have slammed into me. Shit, I think my car's totaled."

"Were you wearing your seat belt?"

"I usually do, but I was just going to the mall."

"I'm glad that you usually do, but usually isn't often enough, as I'm sure you realize now." As George started to nod his head, I said quickly, "You mustn't move your head, or any other part of your anatomy either. Got it?"

"I guess."

I turned to Stan Portizski, the FPD officer who was gathering information from a bystander. "Stan, could you get one of the crew members from the other car to help me? I need to do a standing takedown."

Stan walked over to the hatchback and replaced Bob Fiorella, who walked back to my patient and me. "Good timing, Joan. We're just about done with the other driver."

"Fuckin' asshole broad," George muttered. "Just look at my car."

"Collar bag, longboard, and the works, Joan?"

"Yup, thanks, Bob." He soon returned with a long backboard, head-immobilizing blocks, and the bag full of cervical collars, straps, and tape. "I think a 'medium' collar will do nicely," I told him. He pulled out the correct size of collar and assembled it for use.

"I'm afraid this isn't designed for comfort," I said to George as Bob fastened the hard plastic collar around his neck. "It's to remind you not to move your head at all."

I saw Stephanie, Nick, and Stan start to slide the woman driver from her car onto another longboard. They would be busy for another few minutes. I needed a third person to do the standing takedown, so I asked a tall, muscular bystander if he would help us.

"Sure, lady. What do you need me to do?"

"What's your name?" I asked.

"Tom."

"Thanks for your help, Tom. Bob will be on one side of George and you on the other," I explained, "while I hold his head." Bob stood the board up on its end, slid it between George and me, up between my arms, and braced the bottom of it with his foot. I was now holding George's head with my arms around the board.

Bob positioned himself facing and in front of George, just to his left. He slid his left hand between George's body and left arm and grabbed a handhold high on the left side of the longboard. "I need you to do exactly what I did, on your side," Bob said to Tom. Bob watched Tom comply, then said, "That's great." Tom now understood that he and Bob were supporting George, each with a forearm high under one of the patient's arms. "Now, hold your side of the board, about waist level, with your other hand."

While Tom got his hands into position, I spoke to our patient. "George, I need you to trust us. We're going to lower you down to the ground. It's going to feel weird, but I promise that we won't drop you."

"Can't I just sit down? I'm not really hurt, you know."

"I understand. But we don't want to take any chances with your neck or spine and this is the best way. If you just relax and let us do our job, that will be the best way to help."

"Okay. If you insist, then go for it," George said.

"Now," Bob explained to Tom, "just walk forward, bend your knees, not your back, and lower the board slowly the way I do. Joan, on your count."

"One, two, three." As Tom and Bob lowered the board from vertical to horizontal, I guided my hands around George's head so that I never lost head stabilization. It took only a few moments until George was lying flat on the board, on the pavement. Tom helped Bob with head immobilization and strapping so that, in less than three minutes, George was firmly affixed to the longboard.

"What about my car?" he said. "What will they do with it?"

"The police will have it towed," I explained. "When you're done at the hospital you can call them and find out where. For right now, let's not worry about your car."

"Yeah, but I've had it for only a month. I just got it new tires, a new battery, shocks . . ."

"Let your insurance company worry about the car."

"Not my insurance company, that broad's insurance company. The whole accident was such bullshit."

Tom and Bob lifted the board and carried George toward the rig. Stephanie and Nick were waiting behind the rig with their stretcher, because it is easier to put a boarded patient onto the crew bench first, before the gurney is loaded.

As the two men began to lift the board into the rig, the woman yelled, "Listen mister. This accident was all your fault. I hope you know that I'm going to sue the daylights out of you."

"Fuck you, lady, it was all *your* fault. You can't just go charging through a damn full stop like you did."

"I'll thank you not to use that language with me, you idiot. Just because . . ."

"Well la-dee-dah, Miss Clean Mouth. I'll use any fuckin' language I want."

"Folks," Stephanie said loudly, "let's let your insurance companies and the police sort this out. You two just calm down."

As Bob and Tom lifted George into the rig, I asked Stephanie, "How is she?"

"She's probably fine. All this," she pointed to the KED, head immobilization, and strapping, "is just precautionary. Yours?"

"Neck pain and a little dizziness. Probably nothing, too, but he broke the windshield with his head. Not a mark on him, though."

"No seat belt?"

"No seat belt."

Once George was secured to the bench, the crew lifted the woman into the rig. Stephanie and I each took a set of vitals and Nick got a blanket for each patient. "Oxygen?" he asked Stephanie.

"None of that shit for me," George bellowed. "You're not putting one of those masks over my face."

"Me either," the young woman said.

"Listen, lady," George continued, "you better wear that oxygen mask. I don't want you givin' me any shit that you were hurt by my car."

"I *was* hurt by your car, Mr. Foul Mouth," the woman said. "They say I might have a neck injury. You slammed into me. . . ."

George interrupted. "Put an oxygen mask in her face, just to shut her the hell up."

"Mind your own business," the girl said. "I'll decide about the oxygen myself."

"Folks," I said firmly, "will you both *please* be quiet and let us do our jobs."

"Fine," they said simultaneously, "but no oxygen."

I looked at Stephanie and we both nodded. Neither patient would suffer from the lack of oxygen. "Okay, no oxygen. Nick," I yelled to our driver, "give us a nice and easy ride to FGH."

I pulled the PCR box from its holder and began to take down George's name and address. At the same time, Stephanie was gathering information from her patient.

"Rosemarie," she was saying to the woman. "Would you please spell your last name."

"Brittenhausen. B-R-I-T-T-E-N-H-A-U-S-E-N."

"Hey," George stopped answering my questions and said, "wait a minute, lady. Did you go to Fairfax High? Graduate about four years ago?"

"Yes, why?"

"I'm George Fowler. We were on the same team in Chem lab."

"You're kidding. George Fowler. I remember you. You were voted 'The guy we'd most like to get trapped on a desert island with.' "

Stephanie interrupted. "Rosemarie, would you tell me your address and answer a few more questions?"

Rosemarie answered all of Stephanie's questions while I finished with George. Then Rosemarie called, "Hey, George, I can't turn my head with it strapped to this thing. Are you badly hurt?" Her voice was filled with genuine concern.

"I can't turn either, but I think I'm fine. Just a little scrambled. How about you? How's your neck?"

"I think it's okay. They just want to protect me. What have you been doing since graduation?"

"I'm a computer accounting clerk for the moment, but I hate my job. I'm thinking of taking a programming course at Fairfax Community College. I work for an asshole . . . Excuse me. I work for a turkey at a firm that manufactures plastic bowls and stuff. What about you?"

The rest of the way to the hospital, George and Rosemarie continued to catch up on their lives since Fairfax High. As we pulled into the ambulance bay, George said, "You know, maybe after we're done here, we could get together. Have dinner. You know. Catch up on old times."

"Yeah, maybe. But we might be in different parts of the emergency room. We might not see each other again today. Why don't you call me when you get home? I'm in the book. B-R-I-T-T-E-N-H-A-U-S-E-N."

"Great, I'll do that."

We delivered our patients to different cubicles. As Stephanie and I did our paperwork, we shook our heads. "Love does strike in the most amazing places," she said.

"Certainly does."

○ ○ ○

JACK MCCAFFREY IS one of the shiest, quietest people I have ever known. When we're on duty together, he usually just sits in the corner of the sofa in the crew room and watches the TV set. He doesn't seem to care what's on, he just watches. When it's mealtime, he takes his sandwich out of the refrigerator, gets a Diet Pepsi from the soda machine, sits at the kitchen table, and eats, then returns to the TV. When someone asks him a question, he responds with as few words as possible. Except when he's with a patient.

Annie Blake was an eleven-year-old girl who had fallen down a flight of stairs and had broken the lower part of her left leg. She had also injured her back. She screamed with pain as we splinted her leg and again as we logrolled her onto a backboard. We talked to her and tried to calm her as we worked to immobilize her as fast as possible, but she was crying with pain and fear as we placed her on a stretcher and loaded her into the ambulance.

Inside the ambulance, I quickly obtained a second set of vitals and we started to roll toward the hospital. Jack began to talk to her.

"What school do you go to?" he asked.

"George Washington," she sobbed.

"Are you sure that's not Benjamin Franklin? I've always thought that all those revolutionary guys were really the same person," Jack said.

"No, it isn't. It's George Washington."

"Isn't he the one who flew the kite in the storm? Almost killed himself, you know. What kind of nut flies a kite in a storm? With a key on it, no less."

"That was Benjamin Franklin."

"Right."

"I go to George Washington School, not Benjamin Franklin," Annie insisted, still whimpering.

"Listen," Jack said, "since you obviously know so much about George Washington, you must know that he was born in a log cabin and walked to school in the snow."

"That was Abraham Lincoln, not George Washington," Annie insisted, no longer crying.

"Yeah, yeah, I knew that," Jack said. "He was the one who wrote the Declaration of Independence."

"That was Thomas Jefferson," Annie said exasperated.

"Right. He was the one who chopped down the cherry tree."

"That was George Washington," Annie said.

"George Washington. That's what I said."

As the ambulance pulled into the hospital, Annie was smiling, having, for the moment, forgotten her pain and fear.

When we left the hospital, I complemented Jack on his ability to make Annie forget her pain, if only for a few minutes. "You were terrific," I said. "You really had her going."

"Yeah," Jack said. That was the last word he uttered on the subject. When we returned to headquarters he walked quietly into the TV room, turned on the set, and watched for the rest of our shift, in silence.

○ ○ ○

AND SOME PATIENTS just make us angry.

The tones went off.

"Fairfax Police to the ambulance corps. A full crew is needed for an automobile accident with injuries. Route 10 near Elm."

I called in and drove to the scene. When I pulled up at the scene I was amazed that anyone had survived. The car was in two pieces, about ten feet apart. The front end that ended abruptly just behind the driver's seat was against a tree. The rear section was upside down in a ditch. The driver was lying in the long grass with Will McAndrews, a Fairfax policeman, leaning over him.

"How is he?" I asked.

"He's doing fine. He says he's all right, but I want him fully immobilized and transported." I was surprised at Will's reaction. Normally, the police wait for us to decide how best to treat the patient.

"Is he complaining of any neck or back pain?"

"No." Will was acting very strangely, but I disregarded it as I started my survey.

I assessed the young man and found that, amazingly enough, he seemed uninjured. The rest of the crew arrived in the ambulance and, as Will had requested, we did a full immobilization, transferred our patient to the stretcher, and lifted him into the rig.

As I started to climb in behind the patient, Will pulled me aside. "I think you should see this," he said as he handed me a crumpled piece of paper. "I found it in his hand."

As I read the block printing, I realized that it was a long, rambling suicide note. "I don't understand," I said. "Do you think he drove into that tree on purpose?"

"Not entirely," Will said through gritted teeth. "Before you arrived, he told me that he had loosened the lug nuts on all the wheels of his car. When one of the wheels finally became loose enough, he lost control of the car. It's a miracle he didn't run head-on into another car instead of a tree. I've phoned ahead and the hospital will hold him there until we get a sergeant and a shrink down there."

"Holy shit," I muttered, picturing the accident that he might have caused. "And he walked away . . ." I looked at the two pieces of the car " . . . from that. And there are so many innocent ones whom we can't save. There's no justice."

I like to feel that I treat all my patients with equal enthusiasm, but I could not in this case. Much to the surprise of the rest of the crew, I made no effort to be civil to him, I made no small talk.

After we transferred our patient to the care of the ER staff, I told the rest of the crew what I had learned. We were all unusually quiet as we drove back to the center of town.

○ ○ ○

I WAS ON duty one afternoon, sitting in the headquarters kitchen with Dave Hancock, Stephanie DiMartino, and Sam Middleton, drinking stale coffee and waiting for a call.

"You know that Ed and I are writing a book," I said, "so I'm always interested in the weird things that happen. Got any stories?"

Dave started. "Okay. I can tell you one, Joan. Sam and I were on duty one midnight about two months ago. The police called and dispatched us to the scene of one of those life-call pendant calls. You know, 'I've fallen and I can't get up.' " He stopped.

"And . . ." I prompted.

"Well, we got no answer when we knocked on the front door. We tried the back door and the garage. Nothing. So the cop had the police dispatcher use the call-back number, but no one answered the phone."

"Amazing. A real call," I said. We get so many false alarms from those pendants that it's unusual to have a real emergency call come in that way.

"Looked like it. So, we had no choice. The cop, Sam, and I had to get into the house. We decided that the garage door was the easiest to break into. The cop used the butt of his gun and pounded on the garage window. Smashed up the window and part of the door pretty good. As we ran into the house, I was sure we'd find someone out on the floor."

Dave warmed up to his tale. "So we walked through the kitchen, yelling, 'Hello, hello there. Ambulance.' All the lights were on, the teapot was whistling, but there was no answer. We looked into each room on the ground floor and found nothing. So we went upstairs and looked into each bedroom. Still nothing. Finally we went through the master bedroom and into the little bathroom. There she was, an elderly lady, sitting, casual as you please, on the john, sound asleep."

"I remember that one," Sam said, laughing. "I'm still wondering whether we'll be sued for the cost of fixing the garage door."

Dave grinned. "How about the guy who got a small doughnut-shaped weight stuck on his dick." The language is often colorful at headquarters, and I've gotten used to it.

"How?" I asked.

"The how is obvious. And as to the why, I have no idea. I guess he was doing his fuck-ups."

"A few years ago, I had a man with his foreskin stuck in his zipper," I said. "He was the classic combination of incredibly embarrassed and hurting like hell. I was crew chief and I walked in first. The man went crazy when he saw me. He made me wait in the living room while the rest of the crew tried briefly to get him free."

"Any success?" Sam asked, his hands clutched in his lap.

"Nope, and they didn't take any chances. After about a minute, they wrapped him up and we transported. The man wouldn't have me in the back. He insisted that I drive. When we unloaded him at the ER, I waited in the rig."

"I guess the lesson is, 'Always wear underwear,' " Sam said.

"I also remember the time when Sam had that asthma attack. It went on for days," Dave continued. "He probably shouldn't have been riding, but try to tell him anything." He looked at Sam and shrugged.

"I wasn't contagious," Sam argued. "I was just exhausted."

"Anyway, we arrived at the home of a tiny little man who was having chest pains. We surveyed him and got ready to transport. We needed a set of vitals, so Sam wrapped the BP cuff around the guy's arm and started to pump. He couldn't hear a thing over the sound of his own wheezing. . . ."

Sam continued the story. "So I handed the stethoscope to Dave. He looks at the BP gauge and fumbles in his pocket for his glasses. Sorry, Sam, he tells me. I can't see a thing without my glasses.

"You should have seen the look on that guy's face. He's got one guy who can't hear and one who can't see. I think if he could've he'd have called another ambulance."

"Then, of course," Dave reminded me, "there was the night the rig got stolen."

Stephanie was relatively new to the squad. "The rig got stolen?"

I think I've told this story 50 times, but I still enjoy telling it. "We got to Fairfax General about two A.M. and delivered our patient. I don't even remember what the call was about. We left the rig running in the ambulance bay, as we always do, while Ed and I changed the linen and Fred did the paperwork."

"Stephanie," Dave said, "you've met Fred Stevens, but you may never have run into his practical joking."

"Is he the one with the filthy mouth?"

"That's Fred."

"So Ed and I finished the stretcher and wheeled it out to the rig. We all but lifted it into empty air. No rig."

"You're kidding," Stephanie said, sipping from a cup of cold coffee.

"Ed and I walked back into the emergency room and asked Fred where he stashed the ambulance. We assumed that he was just kidding around, but he looked at us blankly. 'What do you mean the rig's missing?' he said. 'I didn't move anything. You're shittin' me.'

"Finally we convinced Fred that this was no joke by walking him out to the bay. No rig."

"What had happened?" Stephanie asked. "Who would steal a big orange and white ambulance?"

"We found out later that a patient had come into the emergency room, drunk, with a cut on his head from a minor auto accident. Once he was bandaged, he wanted to go home and, because his car was smashed up, he 'borrowed' the ambulance. The key was in it, and it was running, so off he went."

"So what did you do?"

"First we called the cops. It took a full minute before they understood that we were serious. When a cop arrived at the hospital, we walked out into the bay to show him where the rig had been. While we were talking, Ed glanced out toward the street and saw the ambulance drive by, heading toward Prescott."

"You gotta be kidding."

"Nope. 'There it goes,' Ed yelled and the cop took off like a bat. Half an hour later, seven police cars had the rig stopped and surrounded. The poor man staggered out of the rig, not sure what all the fuss was about."

"I recall that it took all night to get the rig back from the police," Dave said. "Fortunately, we have two others." He paused. "Remember this one, Sam? About a year ago, we had a weird one. I remember it had been a busy morning. We had already responded to a three-car accident on the southbound parkway. No one had been hurt, but as we tried to return to headquarters we had gotten tied up in commuter traffic. Patiently, because we had no place else to go, we waited while the two trucks removed the automobile carcasses and the police got the traffic sorted out."

"I remember that one," Sam said. "Don't brag about your patience, however. You were a pain in the ass. 'My coffee. I haven't had my coffee.' "

"We had been back at headquarters for only half an hour when we received a call for another accident, just north of the previous one. As we approached the scene, we saw a police car pull up behind a van stopped in the center lane of the parkway. Leaving the lights on his car flashing, the cop jumped out and began to direct traffic around the accident site."

"Yeah," Sam continued, "I pulled in behind the police car and, leaving all our lights flashing to warn other drivers, Dave and I went around to the driver's side of the van. All the windows were closed and the engine was running."

Dave went on. "We saw a man slumped over the wheel, unconscious, and we tried to open the doors. I leaned around so I could see the man's face through the windshield. 'Sir,' I called, 'are you okay. Can you open your door for us?' "

Dave started to chuckle. "Groggily, the man raised his head. Obviously disoriented, he still managed to reach around and open the driver's door. Before he could move anymore, I reached in and supported his head. 'Sir,' I said, quietly, 'what happened?'

" 'I have no idea,' he answered. 'Who the hell are you?' "

Sam said, "While Dave checked the patient, I walked around the car. There was no damage. No damage at all."

Dave continued the story. "I told the man my name, then asked him again what had happened. 'Did you have an accident?' I asked. He said he didn't know. He said he had no pains, no nothing.

" 'So what's the last thing you remember?' I asked.

" 'I was stuck in traffic. I think there was an accident up ahead. I'm kind of groggy, I'm afraid. I've been driving all night.'

"Suddenly, I understood. 'Is it possible you fell asleep while your car was stopped in the traffic jam?' "

Dave shook his head slowly. "And that was exactly what had happened. He was stuck there so long that he must have just fallen asleep. Five minutes later, when we were sure he was unhurt, we warned him to get some shut-eye immediately and sent him on his way. Weird, no?"

HEADQUARTERS

AS YOU ALREADY know, we at FVAC try to have a full crew of at least three on duty at all times. Unfortunately, with the increase in two-income families, it has become harder and harder to find people who are available on weekdays. Even on weekends, now, we are having trouble getting a full crew who can be on duty at headquarters.

FVAC responds to about 1,500 calls a year, or about four calls a day. Because a call usually lasts about an hour, you can see that during a six-hour shift, most of the time is spent sitting and waiting. To lure crews and off-duty personnel to headquarters, we try to keep our building as pleasant as possible. Let me take you on a tour.

One side of the building is entirely occupied by the garage. There is room for three ambulances. The first- and second-due rigs, usually 45–01 and -02, are parked side by side just behind the two big electric doors. The third rig, usually 45–03, is parked just behind 45–01.

Behind 45–02 is a huge closet filled with first-aid supplies, extra linen, and a cascade system, three enormous oxygen bottles that we use to refill the smaller portable tanks we carry on the ambulance. The closet is further cluttered with wheelchairs, crutches, and various sick-room supplies that we lend to community members free of charge.

Next to the garage is a small dispatcher's area, containing the Fairfax police radio, a scanner, and a CB radio. Just beyond is the eat-in kitchen, the center of activity at FVAC. During the day there are usually several members sitting around, gossiping, checking out the contents of the large refrigerator, and drinking stale coffee.

The 6 P.M. to midnight shifts are the only ones consistently filled by regular crews, many of whom have ridden together for many years. In some crews each member brings his own dinner, in some one member, on a rotating basis, brings dinner for the entire crew.

Only one has Greg. You've already met Greg Horvath, one of our dispatchers. Although he frequently dispatches during the day, he also rides 6 P.M. to midnight each Wednesday. Because he's retired and loves to cook, everyone chips in for the cost of the ingredients, and he prepares dinner each week. He used to prepare enough for himself, his wife, and the crew of four. Now, so many people "drop in" around dinnertime each Wednesday that he prepares enough for a dozen. And he loves it.

He usually prepares the meal at home, then brings it to headquarters at around 5:30. The crew arrives just before six and dinner's usually ready by about 6:15, when Greg's wife arrives to share the goodies. In addition to the quality of the food, there is another advantage to Greg's cooking. If a call comes in at dinnertime, and Murphy's Law says it usually will, Greg stays behind, works the radio, and keeps dinner warm.

I particularly enjoy Greg's chili. When I asked him whether I could use his recipe in this book, he was delighted. A few days later, I found the following note in my corps mailbox:

Dear Reader,

Because of the confined quarters in the back of the rig, EMTs are concerned about the type of food they consume. Obviously garlic and onions are no-no's and you would think that crews would also be wary of anything that contains beans. Therefore, a recipe for chili might cause eyebrows to be raised.

The following chili is pretty much "report free," however, due to the "magic" preparation of the beans. I usually make the chili in advance, then bring it to headquarters. While I prepare the corn bread, I reheat the chili in the microwave, a pot, or a large frying pan. Both the chili and the corn bread can be kept warm if Wednesday dinner is interrupted by an ambulance call.

Greg's User-Friendly No Back-talk Chili

Serves 4 to 5 people (although I usually double the recipe to feed the people who accidentally "drop in" at mealtime).

1 pound dried beans (any kind desired)
1 pound ground beef, turkey, or chicken
2 quarts spaghetti sauce
One package chili mix
Garlic and/or onion powder to taste
Olives, nacho chips, cheddar or jalapeño cheese for garnish
Tabasco for those who want extra heat

Soak beans overnight and discard the water.
Cook beans until tender according to the instructions on the package and again discard the water.
Brown the meat and add sauce, chili mix, and garlic and/or onion powder and simmer, tasting frequently (that's the fun part).
Garnish as desired.
If you have the time, refrigerate for the next day's use to allow flavors to blend. Add a bit of water at reheating time if desired.
Preparation of the beans is obviously a little time-consuming. You can prepare larger quantities with the above formula as a basis, and freeze the beans for future use.

Preparation time after cooking the beans is about 15 minutes.

30-Minute Corn Bread

1 ½ cups cornmeal
½ cup flour
½ cup sugar
2 teaspoons baking powder
1 teaspoon salt
1 teaspoon baking soda
½ cup oil—I use the kind with the lowest cholesterol
1 ½ cups low-fat milk
1 teaspoon vanilla
2 eggs beaten (I use the equivalent amount of egg substitute)

Heat oven to 425 degrees.
Grease the bottom and sides of a 9″ × 14″ baking pan with margarine or butter. I use a pan that's nonstick coated so I don't bother with grease.
Mix dry ingredients in a large bowl.
Add the remaining ingredients and pour the resulting batter into the baking pan.
Bake in center of the oven for 15 minutes.
The top of the corn bread will be golden brown when finished. It comes out very flat but moist. It's delicious directly from the oven and wonderful cut into bread-sized pieces and popped into the toaster.

Last year, on Greg's birthday, we all got him a cake. In addition, four people got him the same gag gift, a bottle of Beano, a brand-name product that eliminates the gaseous effects of such foods as broccoli, Brussels sprouts, and beans.

Beyond the kitchen is the TV room. It's furnished like a living room, with sofas and chairs that have been bought or donated over the years. The furniture must be replaced frequently because it gets a lot of use. We don't really care about the decor, but we always have a good large-screen color TV to lure members to headquarters. We get every possible channel, so the TV is usually on from early morning to midnight, when the night shift leaves. We sometimes have World Series or Super Bowl parties with food and drinks, but never alcohol.

Sometimes night-shift riders choose to sleep over in one of our two small bedrooms, each of which has two single beds. At other times, crew members ride from home, as Ed and I usually do, and respond to the scene or to headquarters if a call comes in. In the winter, if the weather is bad, of course, we all ride from headquarters.

Ed and I have ridden together from headquarters, and it really is a drag that the corps has only single beds. I'm told that, years ago, single beds didn't keep two members of nearby Prescott Volunteer Rescue Squad from enjoying some time together in their headquarters' back bedroom. Unfortunately, they were married, but not to each other, at the time.

No one would have been aware of what was going on, except for Hugh Washington's scanner. It was about 1 A.M. and Hugh was at home, not yet in bed. He heard the police dispatched to a possible rollover and, because he was the driver on the crew that night, he decided to go to Prescott headquarters in case the rig was needed. When he arrived in the building, the noises coming from the bedroom were unmistakable. When the tones went off a moment later, the couple, buttoning and zipping, ran from the bedroom. After the call, they were both so embarrassed that they left the squad.

The largest room in our headquarters is our meeting- and classroom. Once a month there is a general membership meeting at which items of interest to the entire corps are discussed. We hear a report from our captain about the day-to-day occurrences of the past month and from the board chairperson about the operations and finances of the corps. Because emergency medicine is constantly evolving, at the end of each meeting we have a training session, detailing the use of new equipment and procedures.

In addition to meetings, the room is used for CPR, first-aid, driver training, and infection control classes. From time to time, we also have held 110-hour EMT courses in-house.

Besides two bathrooms, the only other room in our building is the small office in back of the meeting room. It contains a desk and chair, a typewriter, a copier, a computer with spread sheet and word processing capabilities, and a dozen file cabinets. This room not only allows people to do office-type work while on duty, it also gives members a private place to conduct business.

Currently, we are hoping to further expand our building and repave our 20-car parking area.

SEVEN

LINDA CONTINI HAD been divorced for two years. She was pretty, with long blond hair and large mahogany-brown eyes, and had been successful at combatting her tendency to put on weight in places where she didn't want extra weight. As a symbol of her new life, she had tried to give up smoking several times, but each time she stopped she began to gain weight. So each time she went back to cigarettes.

At first, being twenty-seven and single again had meant a series of very short, nonserious relationships. There was no shortage of men and, unwilling to form close bonds, she had her share of one-night stands and brief, nonthreatening flings. All she had wanted were more "notches on her garter belt."

Then she met Jonathan and soon after, Carlo. Each man wanted something more from her than casual sex. Linda found herself spending a lot of time with each of them, more than she really wanted to.

The weekend had been particularly full but exhausting. She had spent Saturday night with Jonathan, who had asked her to marry him. She had quickly refused, realizing that Jonathan was not someone she wanted to spend the rest of her life with. No one was.

This morning, she had walked along the path around the reservoir with Carlo. They had marveled at the autumn palette of maple-oranges, birch-yellows, sumac-reds, and oak-browns on the steep mountain slopes to the east, and the stillness of the surface of the water. They had picnicked on sandwiches they had brought along, and then had spent much of the quiet Sunday afternoon feeding the ever-present hordes of Canada geese.

Carlo had wanted to spend the evening with her, but as much as she enjoyed being with him, Linda had wanted to relax at home alone. Since her divorce she had learned to enjoy having time alone—all to herself—and would not allow anyone to take that time away from her, especially Carlo, who was getting much too serious.

It was late evening, and Linda was stretched out on her unmade bed, reading one of the wonderfully predictable romance novels that she loved. An ashtray rested on the sheet next to her as she smoked her last cigarette of the day. She realized that she was having trouble concentrating on the story, so she reread the sentence that she had just read. She wasn't aware of her eyelids flickering, then closing.

As her arms relaxed, her hands fell to her sides and the book dropped softly onto her chest. The cigarette remained between the fingers of her right hand, the glowing end now pressed against the sheet. A wisp of smoke arose from the bed.

As Linda slept, the cigarette burned through the sheet and into the mattress. Although neither the sheet nor the ticking actually caught fire, the mattress stuffing smoldered for a while. Finally the burning stopped and the smoke in the room dissipated.

"Fairfax police to all Fairfax Ambulance pagers and home units. A full crew is needed to respond to 444 Lyndon Place for an unconscious female."

It was early Monday morning and I was contemplating the dubious joys of being a single father. I had just gotten the kids off to school and was finally relaxing and having breakfast. I had chewed only a few more mouthfuls when the voice intoned the message a second time.

Oh, well, I thought. Lyndon Place is only about a two- to three-minute drive from my house. The rest of my breakfast will have to wait. I grabbed my radio and keyed the mike.

"45–22 to Fairfax PD."

"Fairfax PD on."

"I'll respond to the scene. Get someone to pick up the rig and two additional members if possible."

"10–4, Ed."

"Is there an officer at the scene?"

"No, negative, but there's a car en route."

Every occupation has its own lingo. In our local police jargon, it's never "yes" or "no" but "yeah, affirmative" or "no, negative."

"10–4, Fairfax PD. Advise me of who will be responding and the ETA of the rig. 45–22 clear."

I pulled up to the house with my green light blinking just as Fairfax police car 317 stopped in the driveway with its red lights flashing. Officer Merve Berkowitz and I were met outside by a woman in her fifties.

"I can't wake my daughter up," she frantically cried.

"What happened?" I asked as we approached the house.

The woman hurried along the front walk, puffing as she ran. "I live just down the street. I tried to call my daughter this morning, but she didn't answer, so I came over. I can't wake her up." Her voice rose until, as we neared the front door, she was nearly shrieking.

We entered the front room. "Do you smell something?" Merve asked, twitching his nose.

"It smells smoky," I admitted, "but there's no obvious smoke in the air."

Merve keyed his mike. "317 to headquarters."

"Headquarters on."

"Better get the fire department over here for a smoke investigation."

"10–4, 317."

The older woman led us down a long hallway and into a sparsely furnished bedroom. Nothing in the room appeared unusual. Except for the gray color of her face, the girl on the bed seemed to be sleeping, her long blond hair spread around her head like a soft cloud.

As a matter of routine, I reached toward the girl's neck to check her carotid pulse, knowing what I would find. Her skin was already cold. I tried to lift one arm, but her pulseless body was already beginning to stiffen. Purple bruises had formed on the lower surface of her upper and lower arms.

I reached for my radio, thinking of the ambulance speeding to the scene.

"45–22 to 45–01."

"01 is on."

"Proceed with caution. This is a 10–45."

"10–4, Ed."

10–45, the code for an obvious death. As EMTs we can't "pronounce"—declare someone dead. Our CPR protocols state, however, that there are indicators of obvious death. Rigor mortis, a stiffening of the body that begins long after death, and dependent lividity, the gravity-caused pooling of the blood in the lowest areas of the body, are two of those indicators. I did not start CPR.

I will always remember my last image of Linda, the ashtray on the bed and the small black hole in the sheet.

The medical examiner later reported that Linda had died of smoke inhalation.

○ ○ ○

"FAIRFAX POLICE TO Fairfax Ambulance," the dispatcher said, breathlessly. "Dispatch an ambulance to 756 Oak Hill for a child turning blue. Respond code 3."

"10–4, ambulance responding." Judy Lloyd dropped the mike on the counter and ran toward the driver's side of the rig.

"Oh, shit," I muttered, dashing toward the passenger door, "a child not breathing." *At least we're a strong crew,* I thought. Joan's daughter Judy is a great EMT and Marge Talbot is solid in a crisis.

Marge leapt into the back and slammed the door. Lights flashing and siren screaming, we sped toward Oak Hill. In the back of the rig, heedless of the need for a seat belt,

Marge scrambled around, grabbing the pediatric bag and oxygen equipment. "Any idea of the age of the child?" she yelled.

I keyed the mike and spoke loudly over the siren. "45–01 to Fairfax Police."

"PD on."

"Any details? Age of the child? Downtime?" I was asking for the length of time since the child had become unconscious.

"Nothing," Mark Thomas answered. "The woman yelled that her child was turning blue, gave the address, and hung up. We're trying to call back, but we're not getting an answer."

"10–4."

Three minutes after the call came in, we pulled into the driveway and jumped from the rig. The front door was open. "Fairfax Ambulance," Judy yelled.

"Out here."

We ran through the house and out the back door. A woman was holding a snuffling two-year-old girl, thumb stuffed firmly into her mouth. "She's turning blue," the woman said, her voice quavering, "and her feet are all swollen. I don't know what's wrong."

Three EMTs heaved a collective sigh of relief. The child wasn't in respiratory arrest. "When did this start?" Judy asked.

"Melanie was playing in the pool." She motioned toward a shallow kiddy pool. Her hand shook as she pointed. "I took her out, dried her off, and put on a dry diaper. Then I noticed that her feet were swelling and her legs were turning blue, so I called you. That was about five minutes ago."

The woman lifted one of Melanie's legs. "Look." The child's foot was obviously swollen, and her leg was the blue color that indicated cyanosis, lack of oxygen in the blood of the child's leg. The other leg looked the same, the bluish color extending up to mid-thigh.

"We'll take good care of Melanie, Mrs. . . ."

"Hanover, Maria Hanover. What's wrong with her?" Mrs. Hanover's voice was rising.

"We aren't doctors," Judy said, "but she seems to be behaving all right. She's not sleepy or extra active."

"No," Mrs. Hanover said, "she seems fine, except for her legs."

Judy reached out and easily took Melanie from her mother. "Hi, there, Melanie," Judy said, pulling a small stuffed rabbit from the pediatric bag. "Look what I have for you." The squirming child snatched the bunny from Judy's hand, hugged it in one arm, and stuffed her other thumb into her mouth.

"Now, Mrs. Hanover," Judy continued, "let's get Melanie to the hospital. They'll do some tests and find out what's going on. But she seems fine, other than her legs."

"Oh, thank you. She seems so content with you. Thank you so much."

While Judy held Melanie and Marge got information from the mother, I got a quick set of vitals. Then I felt the child's foot for a pedal pulse. The skin was cool and, not unexpectedly, through the puffiness of the foot, I couldn't feel a pulse.

"Okay," I said, "let's transport."

During the seven minutes it took us to drive to the hospital, Melanie's skin slowly returned to normal and I finally found a good pedal pulse.

We arrived at the emergency room, gave a quick report to Carol Bankcroft, one of the ER nurses on duty, and left Mrs. Hanover and Melanie in her care. As Judy did the paperwork and Marge and I made up the stretcher, I heard Mrs. Hanover call, "Ambulance people."

Judy was still writing, so I walked into the cubicle. "What can I do to help?" I asked.

"The doctor doesn't believe me," Mrs. Hanover said.

"Now, Mrs. Hanover," Dr. Margolis said, looking at the child's legs, which now appeared perfectly normal, "that's not it at all." Skeptically, he turned to me. "How did the child's legs look when you arrived?"

I knew how the doctor felt. We get so many panicky parents who have no idea of how to accurately report a medical problem that it's hard to know exactly what to believe. I described the exact condition of Melanie's legs.

"See?" Mrs. Hanover said, triumphantly. "I told you."

Dr. Margolis sighed. "I'm sorry, Mrs. Hanover. It's not that I didn't trust you. I'm sure you can understand."

"Yes, of course. Anyway, what's wrong with Melanie?"

"Thank's Ed," Dr. Margolis said to me. "We'll take it from here." As I left, Dr. Margolis turned to Mrs. Hanover and began asking her a series of questions.

About a week later, Judy showed me a note she had received.

Dear Fairfax Ambulance,

Last Tuesday you came to my daughter's aid. In her twenty-three months she had had no difficulties before, so when her feet swelled and suddenly turned blue, I was so frightened. I can't tell you how much you helped us that day. You all acted with a professionalism that really mattered. You took control when we really needed it.

Melanie is fine now. She was diagnosed as having Raynaud's phenomenon, which may go away with time or stay the same. There is a slight chance it might turn into Raynaud's disease, which is a more serious circulatory problem, but that is unlikely. It looks like she is unusually sensitive to cold, but we can all deal with that.

We'll never forget your help. Melanie is precious to us beyond words. And, by the way, she loves her new bunny.

Maria Hanover

Judy looked at me and smiled. "It's nice when things work out so well," she said.

"And it's nice to know we're appreciated."

"Well," Judy said, "we're terrific. That's why they pay us volunteers the big bucks."

○ ○ ○

IT WAS A bright, sunny Indian summer day, a perfect day for the annual county lifesaving awards ceremony, held this year in a local park. I had received an award the previous year, and this year Joan was very proud to be receiving one for her defibrillation "save" of a few months earlier. We watched EMTs and paramedics from other local rescue squads file onto the platform to receive awards, which were being presented by the county EMS commissioner.

After handing out awards to a rescue-squad crew from our neighboring town, the commissioner stepped down from the platform and Mike Gold, a police officer from the nearby town of Prescott, walked up to the microphone. Joan and I exchanged glances.

Mike, a twenty-seven-year-old officer who always seemed to have a smile on his face, had been a student in one of the EMT courses that we had taught together. He had been one of the first Prescott officers to be trained as an EMT. We knew that he had been in some lifesaving situations himself, and I wondered what he was going to say. Was he receiving an award for something?

Mike began to speak. "I requested that I be allowed to present the next award because it is of special significance to me. . . ."

"325 to Car 706."

"06," Mike responded, wondering what his headquarters wanted from him now.

It was almost the end of his shift and Mike was looking forward to getting home and going for a swim in the pond near his home. His kids would probably be in the water—they usually were on days like this. So far, it had been one of the hottest days of the summer but, thankfully, a quiet one. One last call and he would be off duty.

"706, respond to the end of Spencer Street for a dumping complaint."

"10–4," Mike replied, making a U-turn, "I know the area."

Spencer Street was one of the most isolated streets in Prescott. It ended in a forested area that, because of its remoteness, was a favorite trash dumping area. There wouldn't be much that he could do except check the details and write a report of the incident. The highway department would pick up the trash on its next regular collection day.

As Mike reached the end of Spencer, he saw that an old, rusty refrigerator had been dumped about 25 feet from the road. It looked incongruous, surrounded by wildflowers. Whoever had left it there hadn't even bothered to remove the door, which was closed. Mike realized that he would have to remove it himself before leaving the scene. With the door on, the refrigerator was a dangerous invitation to neighborhood children.

Mike reached down beside the seat of his patrol car and popped the trunk release, then reluctantly got out. He really didn't feel like fighting with rusty hinges in 90-degree heat. He also didn't particularly want to walk through 25 feet of grass and brush. The deer population in this part of town was astronomical because of the adjacent state park. About 75 percent of the Prescott cops had already contracted Lyme disease. In addition, he knew he was allergic to poison ivy, and the rusted copper-colored box seemed to be resting in a field of it.

Well, it's all part of the job, Mike thought as he reached into the trunk of the patrol car for a screwdriver. With a little luck, that would be all he'd need.

He walked through the grass and opened the refrigerator. Having made sure that it was empty, he began to unscrew the upper hinge bolt. Sweat was already running down the sides of his face. Insects buzzed around his face, and he swatted them away.

"Little bast . . . ," he started to say, when he suddenly felt as if a red-hot poker had been plunged into the inside of his lower lip. He spat a bee out of his mouth.

As far as Mike could remember, he had been stung by a bee only once before, as a kid. It had hurt for a while and swelled a little, but that was all. Although his lip began to hurt like hell, he was not particularly concerned. He wondered if the insect-bite swabs in his first-aid kit could be used in the mouth.

He started to walk back to his car. Suddenly the world began to spin and Mike felt that he couldn't breathe. Although it had been less than a minute since the sting, he felt heavier than he had ever been in his life. His legs could not support him.

As an EMT, Mike knew what was happening. Anaphylactic shock—an extreme allergic reaction to the bee sting. Mike knew that there was nothing that he could do for himself. Unless he could get help, he would soon die.

The 25 feet to the patrol car seemed like miles, and Mike had to crawl the last few feet. By the time he managed to get his upper body into the car he was only semiconscious and could hardly speak around a swollen tongue that occupied almost all of his mouth. He reached for the microphone and pressed the send key. All he could say was, "706, 10–13." 10–13, the police code for "officer needs assistance."

I'm dying, he thought. Although Mike could no longer speak, he could hear the police dispatcher repeatedly demand, "325 to 706. What is the nature of the problem?" Soon, even that sound faded out.

Hearing Mike's call, police units from all over the township began to converge on the last known location of his patrol car. "Officer needs assistance" is a code seldom heard in suburbia, and every officer who could move was responding.

Unable to obtain a further response from 706 and unable to determine why Mike had called for assistance, Prescott police headquarters dispatched fire equipment and an ambulance to Spencer Street.

Stan Garth, in car 715, was the first to reach the end of Spencer Street. "I'm at the end of Spencer and the 706 car is here," he said into the radio, "unknown problem. Be advised that 715 is out of the car."

Stan jumped out of the car and found Mike facedown across the front seat of the car. He keyed Mike's radio. "Officer down. I don't think he's breathing. Get an ambulance here fast."

"Prescott Rescue already rolling, 715. ETA one minute."

Stan pulled Mike out of the car, placed him on his back, and placed his cheek next to Mike's mouth. Mike was not breathing. Stan tried to give breaths but couldn't seem to get more than a tiny bit of air into Mike's lungs. He felt for a pulse in Mike's neck and found none.

Stan had just started CPR compressions when Officer Roy Zimmerman arrived on the scene. "I'm having trouble getting air in," Stan said, reassuming his position behind Mike's head.

"Want me to try?" Roy said.

"I've got a good seal. It's like his lungs will only hold a little air. And his mouth is all swollen."

"That rig better get here soon," Roy said as he began chest compressions.

Moments later the Prescott Rescue Squad ambulance pulled up, lights flashing and siren screaming. Paramedic Hugh Washington jumped out of the passenger seat even before EMT Sally Walsh could pull the rig to a stop. At almost the same instant, Paramedic Amy Chen arrived in her own car, having left her four-month-old baby with a neighbor when she heard the call.

"Amy," Hugh said. "Glad you're here. You and Sally get the defibrillator, oxygen duffel . . . You know what we'll need."

"Will do."

Hugh ran over to the police car. "What've we got?"

"I found him half in, half out of the car, in full arrest," Stan said. "I had just begun CPR when Roy arrived. We've been pumping and blowing ever since. Look at his mouth. It's all swollen and I've been having a hard time ventilating. His lungs don't feel right." From the look of Mike's face and mouth, Hugh quickly guessed that Mike was in anaphylactic shock.

"His lungs are probably full of fluid," he said to Stan. "Okay, guys. Stop CPR." Hugh pressed his fingers lightly on Mike's neck and bent over to listen for breathing. He counted to five. "No breathing or pulse. Continue CPR while we get organized."

Amy and Sally arrived with the megaduffel and an oxygen roll. "I'll intubate," Hugh said. "Amy, start a line. Sally, get the monitor set up."

Amy quickly got a large-bore needle into the vein in Mike's arm and started a 1000 cc bag of lactated Ringer's solution. Sally had a little trouble cutting Mike's shirt off, then had to contend with his bullet-proof vest. When his chest was exposed, she took three electrodes from the defibrillator pack and pulled the backing off the adhesive. With Amy's help, she put one pad on the patient's upper right chest, one on his upper left chest, and one on his lower left ribs.

As Amy and Sally worked, Hugh moved Stan out of the way and took over Mike's airway. He set up the laryngoscope and lubricated the endotracheal tube. He quickly slipped the blade of the laryngoscope under Mike's epiglottis and, using the light, passed the endotracheal tube between Mike's vocal cords and into his trachea. Then he inflated the bulb and hooked up the BVM. Now Hugh could ventilate directly into Mike's lungs.

"Sally," Hugh said, "hook up the O_2, then elevate his feet. Amy, get lung sounds as I bag." Hugh squeezed the bag, barely getting any air into Mike's lungs. "Shit, I have so much resistance I'm getting nowhere."

Amy auscultated each of Mike's lungs, using her stethoscope to listen for breath sounds. "Air's moving, but the sounds are really muffled." She moved the diaphragm of the stethoscope to the epigastric area and listened as Hugh squeezed the bag. No air was leaking into Mike's stomach. Amy nodded. All clear so far.

Hugh taped the tube in place and put an oral airway in Mike's mouth to keep him from biting the tube if he awakened. *When he awakens,* Hugh corrected himself.

"What do you see?" Hugh asked Amy, who was checking the screen of the cardiac monitor.

"V-fib," Amy answered. "You want epi?"

Hugh nodded as he squeezed the BVM in rhythm with Roy's compressions. Amy set up 1 mg of 1:10000 epinephrine solution and Hugh introduced it directly into Mike's lungs through the endotracheal tube. The solution would be absorbed directly into the membranes of his lungs, like an inhaler, to reduce the swelling and help open Mike's airway.

Amy again checked the monitor. "Stop compressions." Roy stopped compressing Mike's chest. "I still read coarse V-fib. Let's give that epi a minute to penetrate. Continue CPR while I get the paddles."

Amy pulled out the shocking paddles from the defibrillator and squeezed a big dollop of conducting lubricant on the surface of one. By rubbing the paddles together, she spread the gel on both, then set the power level to 200 joules.

Sally held the diaphragm of the stethoscope over the apex of each of Mike's lungs while Sally again listened as Hugh bagged, the effort rapidly getting easier. "Better. Air's moving better."

Amy pressed the paddles against Mike's chest. "Ready?"

"Go for it," Hugh said.

"Clear back," Amy yelled over the loud tone the machine gave off as it charged. Hugh felt for a pulse in Mike's neck and, finding none, indicated to Amy that he was still pulseless.

Amy pressed the button on each paddle. Mike's entire body jerked for an instant, then was still.

"Still coarse V-fib," Amy said, checking the monitor as the machine recharged. "Clear again."

Again the machine charged, again Hugh checked Mike's neck, and again Amy shocked Mike's heart. She checked the monitor. "Yeah! Looks like we've got a rhythm," Amy yelled. "SVT at about one hundred and thirty."

Sally looked puzzled. She'd run several codes in her year in the squad but hadn't learned all the lingo yet. "What's SVT?"

"Supraventricular tachycardia," Hugh said as he continued to assist Mike's breathing. "A viable rhythm, but very fast. Looks like we've got him back." Hugh quickly guessed Mike's weight at about one hundred and seventy pounds and calculated. "Let's push seventy-five milligrams lidocaine." He looked at Sally. "That's to keep the heart muscle from returning to ventricular fibrillation."

"You mean he's alive?" Roy asked as Amy gave Mike the lidocaine through the already-flowing IV.

"He's still not breathing, but his heart is beating," Hugh said, grinning. "So far, so good. We're going to start another line to give him some more meds, then we'll transport." Amy started a second IV and began a slow lidocaine drip. They finished, lifted Mike onto a longboard, then onto the stretcher.

In the ambulance, Sally checked Mike's wrist. "I've got a radial pulse. Any respirations?"

"He's making the effort," Hugh said. "I get a shallow breath every three or four squeezes."

"Thank God for paramedics," Sally said, thinking of all the surrounding towns that had only EMTs and basic life support rather than advanced life support with paramedics. "Without the meds, he wouldn't have come back. This is one of those cases where EMTs wouldn't have been able to save him. What if he'd been in some other town?" Sally climbed out of the back so she could drive the rig to the hospital.

"They would have done the best they could and transported, code 3," Amy answered. "Let's just be grateful that we were there."

By the time Mike arrived at St. Luke's, he was breathing on his own. He was admitted, stayed for 72 hours, then was discharged.

* * *

" . . . and so it is my great joy to present county lifesaving awards to Prescott police officers Stan Garth and Roy Zimmerman, and to Prescott Rescue Squad volunteer paramedics Hugh Washington and Amy Chen and EMT Sally Walsh . . . for saving my life."

○ ○ ○

ONE THING IS certain in emergency medical work. The unexpected will happen. Just when you have had a long streak of calls involving chest pains, breathing difficulties, insect stings, and febrile seizures, you will find yourself in a situation unlike any that you have ever experienced or anticipated, and for which you are totally unprepared.

We had just started our shift and were checking out the rig, as each crew does on every six-hour shift. I had just pulled the oxygen tank out of the crash bag of 45–01 and had opened the main valve. The pressure in the tank was 1,850 pounds per square inch—enough to last about 45 minutes, and close to the maximum pressure that the tank can hold. I opened the flow valve and heard the gentle hiss of flowing oxygen. I closed the flow valve and pressed the button on the positive pressure/demand valve. A rush of oxygen told me that it, too, was working okay. Suddenly the claxon sounded and the loudspeaker blared.

"Fairfax Police to Fairfax Ambulance."

The police dispatcher's voice had sounded particularly excited. I quickly closed the main valve of the oxygen, bled the line, replaced the tank in the crash bag, and strapped the bag onto its shelf.

I heard Jill Tremonte key the mike. "Ambulance on."

"An ambulance is needed at 1580 Blackberry Hill Road, the Johnstone residence. A child has been attacked by a snake. All I could get was that the snake's still wrapped around him."

Jill's pen almost fell out of her hand as she attempted to jot down the information. "Say again, Fairfax Police."

"We need the ambulance at 1580 Blackberry Hill Road. A child has been attacked by a snake."

"10–4 Fairfax Police. 45–01 is responding to 1580 Blackberry Hill Road for a snake attack," she responded, her voice quavering. "Do you have any additional information?" she asked.

"Negative. The caller hung up before we could get any more information."

We sped down Route 10. I had no idea of what we were going to find when we got to the scene. "A child attacked by a snake? It's wrapped around him?" I muttered as we sped through traffic.

"I know nothing about snakebites, Ed," Jill said, "and I don't want to know. I hate snakes."

"My daughter Arielle just got a pet snake," I said, "but I must admit I've never held it. I'm not afraid of snakes, though, just not eager to make friends."

"Good," Steve Nesbitt yelled from the back of the rig. "If you don't mind snakes, Ed, this one's all yours."

We all have irrational fears. Mine is heights. I have always been terrified that I might have to treat a patient on a high ledge of a building or a cliff. I'm not sure that I would be able to do it. That's the way Jill and Steve were acting about snakes. I guess it's lucky that the snake wasn't on a ledge.

As I thought about it, I realized that the dispatch information did not make sense. Our local snake species don't attack people. They may bite if cornered or stepped on, but they would then try to get away. And, as far as I know, there are no constrictors in the United States. Even if there were, the only constrictor large enough to eat a man is an anaconda, and they live in the Amazon rain forest.

The dispatcher must have been wrong about the snake being wrapped around the patient. Someone must have stepped on or tried to pick up a garter snake or a black rat snake and gotten bitten. The tiny pinpricklike punctures would probably not even require medical treatment although we'd have to transport anyway. "First thing to do for a snakebite," I muttered, "is call poison control."

"The police may have already done that," Jill said.

It must be a simple snakebite, I thought. The worst-case scenario would be a copperhead bite, which could be serious. But copperhead bites are not nearly as dangerous as people think they are. They can cause a lot of local tissue destruction, but they are rarely fatal, and to the best of my knowledge poisonous snakes do not always inject venom when they bite.

I expected to find our patient outside when we arrived at the scene, but there was nobody around. I led the group that walked into the house.

"Hello," I called. "Fairfax Ambulance."

"Up here."

Following the voice, we walked up the stairs and into the bedroom at the end of the hall. All along one wall of the room was a huge glass and wire-mesh enclosure. A teenaged boy was standing in the center of the room frantically pulling at his upper right arm. Wrapped around his arm was a large beige and brown-colored snake. The veins of the boy's arm and hand were distended and his fingers were blue. Tentatively I reached for his hand, took his wrist, and felt for a radial pulse. There was none.

"What happened?" I asked.

"BC hasn't been feeling well for the last few days," he answered.

"BC?"

"Yeah, BC—my boa. Get it? BC for boa constrictor. He bit me yesterday when I tried to pick him up. I was going to bring him to the vet today, but when I reached into his cage, he wrapped himself around my arm and constricted."

Officer Chuck Harding had come in behind us, and he quickly sized up the situation. He keyed his radio.

"305 to headquarters."

"Go ahead 305."

"We need the ACO here ASAP."

Jill looked at me and raised an eyebrow.

"The ACO is the Animal Control Officer," I said, and Jill nodded.

"10–4, 305. I'll dispatch him. But he's on the other side of town. It will be awhile until he can get there."

I knew that we could not wait for the Animal Control Officer. The reptile was cutting off the blood supply to the boy's arm. I wasn't sure whether to try to remove him or transport the boy to the hospital with the snake attached, but we had to do something, and fast. The snake seemed to be as tight as a tourniquet. If it was that tight, removing it could cause the boy to go into shock. But the boy might lose his arm if we didn't remove it. Somehow this situation had not been addressed in my EMT training. I had to make a decision with little to go on.

"Let me try to get it off," I suggested.

The snake was like a three-inch-thick steel coil. Even its head was pressed tightly against the boy's arm. It was impossible to get a grip on any part of it. It stared as I tried to get a finger hold, its tongue rapidly flicking in and out, tasting the air.

"There's no way we can pull it off," I said. "We're going to have to kill it." I had no idea of how we could accomplish that without injuring the boy's arm. I wasn't even sure that killing the snake would make it release its hold.

"No, don't hurt BC," the boy screamed, backing away. "I'll call my mom. She knows all about snakes."

He ran over to the telephone, dialed with his good arm, and after a short conversation held the receiver out to me.

"My mom wants to talk to you."

I took the phone. "Hello, Mrs. Johnstone. This is Ed Herman, with Fairfax Ambulance."

"Hello, Mr. Herman." Her voice sounded calm and competent. "Listen, I did a lot of reading about boas before I allowed Peter to have one as a pet. Boas are tropical, cold-blooded animals. If you cool the snake it will relax. All you have to do is to run cold water over it with the garden hose."

"Okay. It's worth a try," I replied.

I turned to the boy. "Peter, show me where the garden hose is."

The boy led me down the stairs, out the dining room sliding door, down the steps of the deck, to the side of the house. We were followed, at a distance, by the rest of my crew and the officer, none of whom had any idea of what was going on. The hose was attached to a tap and was lying in a heap against the side of the house. I asked Peter to sit down on the ground, removed the hose nozzle, opened the tap and began to pour water over the snake. "Jill, why don't you monitor his radial pulse while I'm cooling the snake," I directed.

Warily, Jill took Peter's wrist, trying to avoid the cold water that was cascading down Peter's shoulder and arm, and trying to keep as much distance as possible between herself and the boa.

After a few minutes, Jill reported, "I feel a pulse."

Peter's hand was still blue, but that could have been partially from the cold water. Now I could see the snake's coils loosening so I reached down and managed to get my fingers around the boa behind his head. Steve grabbed his tail. There was little resistance as we unwound him—all six feet of him—from Peter's arm and put him on the concrete in the shade. I saw Peter flex his fingers and bend his elbow.

I stared at the long reptile stretched lazily on the cool patio. "Was BC this big when you first got him?" I asked Peter.

"No. He was just a baby when I brought him home, two years ago. But snakes grow fast if you feed them a lot. I feed BC as often as he will eat." I thought about Arielle feeding Spike and looked again at the long, thick boa.

Peter reached for BC with his left hand. "Let me take him and put him back in his cage."

None of us argued with him.

Peter returned after a few minutes and we examined him. His upper right arm was red and swollen, but he appeared to have full movement and sensation in his hand and fingers.

His arm would be pretty sore for a while, but there didn't seem to be any major damage. Peter's vital signs were normal. The gamble of removing the snake had paid off. Thank God the boa had not wrapped itself around his neck, I thought.

We called his mother back and related our "success story." After some discussion, Peter's mother decided that Peter didn't need medical attention, so she refused transport for him.

I returned home at the end of my shift to find that my daughter had just gotten home from school. She heard the door slam as I entered the house.

"Hi, Daddy. I'm upstairs feeding Spike. Wanna hold him?"

"I'll be right up. You know, honey, maybe you shouldn't feed him quite so often." I paused. "Remember that poem I used to read to you? The one from *Where the Sidewalk Ends,* about the guy who's being eaten by a boa constrictor."

Arielle laughed. "Sure, I'd forgotten it until now. Why do you ask?"

I just chuckled. "I'll tell you in a minute."

○ ○ ○

THE ACCIDENT HAD occurred on a bad curve of the parkway. As we approached the wreckage, I could see a woman lying in the roadway about 15 or 20 feet from what had, presumably, been a car. How had she gotten there? Had she been pulled out by a well-meaning but ignorant passerby? Had she crawled? Had she been thrown?

I was nervous about my crew. My partner was Tim Babbett, a new probationary member who had, in a short period of time, alienated a lot of corps members. He had recently finished his EMT course at the local community college, but because he was loud, pushy, and kind of weird he had not yet been voted in as a full member. I had more help on the way, but for now it was just the two of us.

I pulled the rig over, told Tim to grab the trauma kit, and walked over to the patient. One glance and I knew that we had to move fast. We had already used seven minutes of the "Golden Hour."

One of the first things EMTs learn is that we have two sometimes contradictory functions, particularly for the seriously injured. Our first job is to stabilize our patient. We stop bleeding, bandage wounds, splint fractures, protect auto accident victims; and our second vitally important function is to transport the patient as quickly as possible to a place where advanced medical care can begin.

We use the term "Golden Hour" to represent the maximum period of time during which we evaluate and stabilize our patient at the scene, prepare him for transport, and speed him to the hospital. In that same hour, the ER staff will again evaluate and treat, X-ray when needed, and relay the victim to the operating room. Our goal is one hour from scene to surgery. If we can meet that goal, we can greatly improve our patient's chance of survival and shorten his recovery time. And that hour was already ticking away.

Our patient was lying on her stomach with her face to the side. There were massive lacerations to what I could see of her face and forehead. Teeth were missing. She must have been thrown from the car and slid along the road for a considerable distance, facedown. Much of her clothing had been torn from her body.

I was overwhelmed. There was so much to do and I had only two hands. As Tim quickly went to the woman's head, I could only hope that he would respond well to the situation.

The woman was screaming that her knees hurt. I couldn't see her knees in the position that she was in, but I was relieved that she was screaming. It meant that she was breathing and had an airway.

Heather and Tom Franks appeared. I glanced at Tim, who seemed to have the woman's airway and breathing under control. I decided to trust him. "Get a longboard, collar, and the stretcher," I said. Someone asked me, "Do you want her on oxygen?"

"Yes, high flow," I answered.

I touched each of her feet, asking her if she could feel my touch.

"Yes," she screamed, "but my knees hurt." Some bone showed through a gash at the top of one foot. At my request, she was able to move the toes on each foot. *So far, so good*, I thought. No obvious spinal injury. I looked up. Tim was calmly and efficiently dressing and bandaging her head injuries. I was very glad he was an aggressive EMT. He just did what needed to be done without being told. I didn't have to divert my attention from what I was doing.

There was so much to be done, so many decisions to be made, all at once. I was faced with my first difficult decision. The woman obviously had trauma to both legs and feet and they should be splinted before she was moved. But she had a possibly severe head injury and, judging from the appearance of the car and her general appearance, she probably had serious internal injuries.

CUPS is the acronym we use to classify the care needs of a patient. Critical, with CPR in progress; Unstable, a patient whose condition is deteriorating; Potentially unstable; or Stable. With a patient whose status is "C" or "U" we *load and go*. With a "P" or an "S" patient, we can *stay and play*.

I made my decision in a matter of seconds. This patient was clearly unstable and she needed advanced care that we couldn't give. We would need to get the patient into the ambulance and rush her to the hospital. "I want to logroll her onto a longboard and I want MAST applied." The military antishock trousers (MAST) would immobilize her legs and feet and help prevent shock.

I examined her legs and pelvis as I cut away her clothing in preparation for applying the MAST. She had numerous lacerations on her legs and feet. The outer layer of skin on her left thigh was almost completely abraded away. Her chest had numerous abrasions. We placed the wooden longboard next to her.

As I was about to consider collar size, Tim said, "I used a trooper to hold her head while I put on a collar. I've got her now and we're ready here. We can turn her on my count." *Great*, I thought. *Just what's needed.* Despite our best efforts, the woman shrieked in pain as we rolled her onto the board.

While applying dressings to her leg and chest injuries, I looked up toward her head. Tim had finished bandaging her facial injuries and was now checking her blood pressure. *Exactly what I need him to do now,* I thought.

"120 over 75," he announced. "Pulse 100, respirations 24 and shallow."

That's fine, I thought. She'd not in too bad a shape.

Heather brought the MAST. "Damn," she said. "Whoever used it last folded it wrong." Heather had to waste precious seconds straightening the MAST and getting it into proper position so we could slide it under our patient. I saw Tim placing the yellow head-immobilizing blocks on either side of the woman's head and readying, but not yet unwinding, tape. He knows to do the head taping last, I realized.

It was difficult sliding the MAST under the injured woman. She was big—almost too big for the trousers. The woman was now naked from the waist down and without clothing to grab, it was difficult to raise her pelvis enough to slide the pants up high enough. With all four of us working, we finally got the pants in place.

"Do you want the MAST inflated?" someone asked.

"No," I responded. "Her BP is okay so far. Let's just strap her down and move."

We quickly immobilized the woman to the longboard and carried her into the ambulance. Inside, I rechecked her BP while a state trooper who had been holding her head asked her questions. Her BP was now about 90 by palpation.

The state trooper was still asking questions. I turned to him. "I'm sorry, Officer, but we have to go. NOW." I leaned through the window into the cab. "Let's roll it, Tom," I said. "Lights and sirens all the way."

The trooper left the rig and we sped down the parkway toward the county trauma center.

"Do you want to inflate the MAST?" Tim asked.

I checked her breathing. Still about 24. Her pulse was rapid but strong. Her fingernails were covered with silver polish, but the skin of her fingers looked normal. I pressed on her knuckle and the skin paled but quickly returned to normal color. I removed her oxygen mask and examined the color of the inside of her lips. Pink. I replaced the oxygen.

"No," I replied to Tim. "Her BP's low, but there are no other signs of shock yet. We'll recheck in a few minutes."

The woman screamed at every bump and curve on the road. She begged to be released from the straps that were tightly securing her to the wooden board, but we couldn't risk additional injury. Tim began talking to the woman, calmly explaining the need for her immobilization. He took her hand. "Squeeze my hand when it hurts," he said softly. "As hard as you can. Go ahead and try to break it." She grasped his hand. While I rechecked the woman's vitals, Tim continued talking to her, reassuring her, encouraging her, telling her that we cared about her.

I stared at him in amazement. Was this the strange guy that people in the corps did not want to ride with? At that moment I could think of very few other EMTs that I would rather have with me on a serious ambulance call.

As we pulled into the ambulance bay, I checked her vitals one last time. Her systolic blood pressure had fallen to 85 and her breathing was more rapid, about 28 breaths per minute. Her pulse felt weaker than it had. We quickly rolled her into the ER and transferred her to the hospital gurney. I relayed all my information to Dr. Margolis, who asked us to inflate the legs of the MAST. After inflation her systolic BP rose to 110.

While Tom and Heather cleaned up the bloody stretcher, I began to write up my PCR. Suddenly I realized that Tim was gone. I glanced into the ER cubicle where our patient was being treated, and there, obviously accepted as part of the trauma team, was Tim, helping to work on the patient. He obviously knew what he was doing in the ER setting as well as at the scene and in the ambulance.

Half an hour later the woman was wheeled to surgery. We radioed our headquarters that we were back in service, and I drove back to the scene of the accident to pick up Tom's car. The wrecked car had been towed away, but as I pulled in behind the Franks's car, I saw that there was still a pool of oil mixed with blood where our patient had been lying. As Tom and Heather walked toward their car, they saw two quarters were lying in the pool. Tom jokingly pointed down and yelled, "Anyone want some money?"

"I don't need two quarters that badly," I laughed as they turned and walked away. I heard Tim climb out of th back of the rig to come around to the passenger side of the cab.

Suddenly, I heard a shout. "Hey, guys, look what I found."

We looked around. Tim was holding up the two oily, bloody quarters.

Heather, Tom, and I looked at one another and shrugged. "Well, he may be a little weird, but he's a great EMT," I said.

TELEVISION

EMTs SOMETIMES GET very frustrated watching TV.

Seat belts. Have you noticed that in most TV shows, the heroes jump into their cars and speed away, never buckling. If the heroes we watch every week would just take five seconds to buckle, those at home might do the same. I'm sure that in those few seconds, the bad guys wouldn't get too much of a head start.

Car ads. A commercial shows an idyllic outdoor scene. There's no sound, just the view of trees and a beautiful waterfall. As the camera pans backward, we become aware that we are in a car. The woman behind the wheel reaches forward and cranks down the window. Suddenly, as the window opens, we hear the thunder of the water, crashing to the pool below. We are supposed to marvel at the interior silence that the car's construction creates.

Automotive silence is an ambulance driver's worst enemy. I've had this experience several times: We're driving the rig code 3, speeding toward the scene of a call with siren wailing. In front of us, there's a driver, plodding along, with no idea that there's an ambulance behind him. I change the siren from wail to yelp. No response. I hit the air horn. Still nothing. Finally, I get on the loudspeaker and say, "Move your car over to the right." If we're lucky, the driver glances in his rearview mirror, sees a large white vehicle with the word AMBULANCE printed on the hood backward so he can read it in his mirror. Startled, he finally pulls over.

That's the problem with a silent car, or one with the radio turned up to full volume and the heater fan on. You have no concept of what else might be on the road with you.

First Aid and CPR. A typical scene from a show about lifeguards: Bikini-clad beauties and men with bodies that women drool over cavort around the beach rescuing swimmers and falling in love.

In one particular episode a man gets trapped beneath an overturned boat filled with water. Quickly and efficiently, the lifeguards pull the man from the craft and attempt to bring him to the surface.

"He's been under too long," someone on the rescue boat says, peering into the water.

As they finally haul the man onto the rescue boat, they notice that his eyes are open. I guess the viewer is supposed to assume that's a sure sign that he's dead.

Now they begin bad CPR by doing a few compressions. No breaths, no checking for pulse or breathing, just a few pounds on the chest. Someone then listens for breathing, or puts an ear to the victim's chest. Hearing no sound, the rescuer shakes his head. "Breathe, damn-you, breathe," someone says. They pound again, still with no results.

The chief lifeguard, the one who's been doing the chest pounding shakes his head again. "No use," he intones, "he's gone."

What hogwash. Not only are the procedures wrong, but a basic principle has been violated. Once you begin CPR, you may not stop unless someone else qualified takes over, the patient revives, or you are just too exhausted to continue and there's no one else who can relieve you. Obviously, in this case, none of these were true.

But he was dead, wasn't he? Also hogwash. People have been revived after prolonged periods of apparent lifelessness. There are many cases of victims, apparently drowned in cold water, having been revived after more than an hour submerged. Even without the benefits of icy water, victims can survive much longer than the four to six minutes we're taught in CPR class. Because of this, only a paramedic or a doctor can pronounce someone dead.

Electrical hazards. TV often shows situations in which an electrocuted person is approached by rescuers before anyone has checked that the power has been turned off or someone "cleverly" lifts a live wire with a wooden pole. Nonsense. You can't do that safely. Even the fire department, with personnel trained in such rescues, waits until the power company guarantees them that the juice has been cut.

I wish that TV shows would just check with a member of their local ambulance corps, fire or police department for the proper procedures. Then members of the TV audience wouldn't become confused and possibly handle their own emergencies incorrectly.

EIGHT

ABOUT TWO YEARS ago, I was aboard a flight that had just taken off from Miami International Airport en route to New York. The man in the seat next to me was a computer salesman from Connecticut who had hardly stopped talking since we left the ground. We talked about flying: how much I hate it and how much he loves it.

"You know, Joan," he said, "flying is so much safer now than even ten years ago. I fly almost every week. My business partner says that I have enough frequent flyer mileage to take me to Jupiter."

I smiled indulgently, wondering how to shut the man up.

"Maybe not enough to do the tour of the great red spot," he laughed at his own humor, "but enough to do the economy package."

Suddenly, a strange, pulsating sound began. The plane began to roll from side to side, like a ship in rough water, and, although I knew that the flight should still be climbing to its cruising altitude, I could feel that it was descending.

"This doesn't feel right," I said, turning to the computer salesman, "and I hate it when the plane does unusual things."

The man's face was white, and his hands gripped the armrests. "So do I," he said.

"Well, I guess everything's okay," I said, looking at the uniformed man taking drink orders from the people in the aisle in front of us. "The flight attendant looks unconcerned."

"This really doesn't feel right. With all my flying, I've never been through anything like this before."

"What good are you?" I protested, not entirely joking. "You said you loved flying. You're supposed to be reassuring me."

"Sorry," he said. "But to be quite honest, I'm scared shitless."

Suddenly the plane's speaker system came alive. The captain's voice, tight and urgent, ordered, "Flight attendants, stow all gear immediately."

Again I looked at the tall, slender, immaculately uniformed young man quickly packing his beverage service gear. Unlike his calm, almost unflappable attitude of a moment before, his face was now pale, strained, and serious.

After a few minutes, the turbulent motion stopped and the plane seemed to have stopped falling. Then the captain spoke again, his voice only slightly more relaxed.

"I apologize for not telling you what's been going on, but we've been a little busy up here," he said. "We've lost one of our engines and we will be making an emergency landing at Orlando in about eighteen minutes." Words of reassurance followed, but as I looked around at the faces of the passengers and flight attendants I could see that everyone was terrified.

"We can fly on only three engines," the computer salesman said. He pulled the information card from the seat pocket in front of him. "Shit," he murmured as he replaced the card.

"What?" I asked.

"We had only two engines to begin with. We're flying on only one now." He swallowed hard and wrapped his hands around the ends of the armrests, his knuckles white.

I swallowed hard, trying to slow my pounding heart. Suddenly I became aware of a disturbance toward the back of the plane and I saw someone hustle past me with an oxygen cylinder.

It was then that my EMT training clicked into gear. I don't know how I would have reacted ten years ago, but now I was trained to act in an emergency. My own feelings ceased to matter. I was on my own form of autopilot.

I carefully got out of my seat and walked up to one of the flight attendants, a sweet young thing who looked no more than sixteen. "I'm an EMT," I told her. "If you need help with any medical problems, I'm in seat fourteen C."

She looked at me with the relieved, grateful expression that I so often see when I identify myself at the scene of an emergency.

"Oh, that's great," she said. "There's a heart patient in back who doesn't seem to be doing well. We're going to put him on oxygen, but we can sure use your help."

I followed her to the back of the plane. In the last aisle seat, I saw a man who appeared to be in his early sixties. Beneath his huge black mustache, his face was pale and he seemed to be struggling to breathe through the oxygen mask that he was clutching to his face. As I slid into the vacant seat next to him, the flight attendant said, "This is Mr. Giovanni."

"Nice to meet you, although not under these circumstances. My name is Joan Lloyd, and I'm an Emergency Medical Technician. The flight attendant tells me that you are having a problem. Can I help?"

"My chest hurts and I can't breathe," he replied. "I have a heart condition."

I reached for his wrist to check his radial pulse. It was somewhat rapid but regular. I watched his chest rise and fall. His breathing rate was fast but within normal limits.

"When did this start?" I asked.

"When the pilot told us that we lost an engine. I'm so scared. How can an engine fall off an airplane?"

The flight attendant, still hovering next to Mr. Giovanni, said, "Sir, the engine didn't fall off. They were just having mechanical problems and the pilot decided to turn it off as a precaution. Flying with an engine turned off is routine."

"I'm sure the flight attendant is right, Mr. Giovanni. You must try to relax. We're in good hands, and I'm sure that the pilot and copilot have the situation completely under control."

The man looked at me suspiciously, not quite believing me. "Are your sure?"

"I'm sure." I didn't know if what I was saying was true or not, but this man was now my patient and my years of training had taken over completely. My only thought was of how to help him. I didn't want to lie to him about the plane, but the line between lying and reassurance was a fine one. And anyway, everything probably was under control now. I began my routine questioning, just as I would have done on a rescue call back home.

"How long have you had a heart condition?"

"Fifteen years."

"Did you take a nitro when the pain started?"

"Yes."

"Did it help?"

"A little. I think I'd like to take another."

"Sure. I can help you, if you'd like." He pulled another tiny pill from the case in his pocket and I helped him put it under his tongue. After a few deep breaths, he released his stranglehold on the armrest.

"Better?" I asked.

"A bit."

"What other medications are you taking?"

"Coumadin and Dilantin."

"Any others?"

"Not that I can think of."

"Mr. Giovanni, do you take birth control pills?"

The man stared at me for a second or two, then grinned. "Naw," he said, "not since I went through menopause, and call me Pat."

Yeah, I said to myself. I knew that I had succeeded in breaking through his fear and tension. I pulled a small pad from my pocketbook and continued collecting information.

There wasn't anything I could do for Pat medically, but there would be an EMS team meeting the plane when it landed, and at least I would be able to give them all the information that they would need about their patient.

Pat and I chatted throughout the rest of the flight, and neither of us noticed the landing. When the plane arrived at the gate, the passengers were asked to remain in their seats so that the emergency medical team could come aboard quickly and remove the man to a waiting ambulance. I went with them as they wheeled the man from the plane, and gave the paramedics the information that I had collected.

"How are you feeling now, sir?" one of the paramedics asked.

"I'm feeling fine. No pain left at all."

"I'm sure it was just a bit of angina," the medic said, "but we'll take you to the hospital to make sure."

"Thanks, Joan," Pat said to me as the paramedic took his blood pressure. "I don't know how I would have made it through without you."

"You would have done just fine," I said, "but I don't know how I would have managed."

"What do you mean?" he asked.

"Okay. I'll 'fess up. I'm terrified of flying and when all hell cut loose up there, I was just as scared as you were. I guess we helped each other through it."

As I stood in the gate area watching the paramedics wheel Pat away, the rest of the passengers began to deplane. The computer salesman walked up to me, still looking shaken.

"What a relief," he said. "I've never been so scared in my life. Did you see all the fire engines that rolled up to the plane after we landed? And look at all the TV cameras. They must all have been expecting a crash."

I had not noticed the landing, the fire engines or the TV cameras until now. As always, on a rescue call, my attention had been so completely focused on my patient that no extraneous factors had registered in my brain.

A couple of days later I called the Orlando hospital to which the man had been taken to find out how he was. He had been treated and released.

○ ○ ○

KEITH AND BECKY Halston had been married for three years and liked to tell friends and family that they were still as much in love as they had been on their honeymoon. A few weeks earlier, Becky had found an advertisement in a catalog, "Learn to Strip for Your Husband." Without Keith's knowledge, she ordered it, hoping she could pull off a birthday surprise. For several days she watched and practiced, working up the nerve to strip for her husband.

Finally, the evening came. The couple came home a bit mellow from a number of glasses of good birthday white wine they had ordered at the restaurant.

"Keith," Becky said, flipping on the bedroom TV, "just relax while I get a surprise ready for you." Keith saw the seductive look in his wife's eyes and, always ready for something exciting, stretched out on the bed.

In the bathroom, Becky took a tight black skirt, a frilly white low-cut blouse and a pair of tiny bikini panties from the linen closet where she had hidden them. "I knew I'd work up the nerve to do this," she whispered to herself. She pulled off the clothes she had worn to the party and stuffed them into the back of the closet. She dressed quickly, dabbed a bit of Opium perfume behind each ear and in a few other strategic places on her body, and opened the bathroom door.

"Turn that thing off, birthday boy," Becky said, lowering her voice and adding a sexy, husky quality. As Keith pressed the off button on the TV's remote control, Becky put a Tijuana Brass tape into the stereo. Moments later, heavy brass music filled the room. Slowly and with increasing bravery, Becky undulated around the bedroom, exposing parts of her body. At one point, barefoot, she stepped up onto the bed and continued her dance. She stepped back onto the floor and slowly pulled off her skirt and blouse. In just her panties, she climbed back onto the bed and teased Keith by rubbing her naked breasts across his chest, always moving out of reach when he grabbed for her.

Finally, she was ready for the pièce de résistance. As erotically as she could, she stepped onto the floor, pulled off her panties, and stepped back onto the bed.

"Wow, baby, you're terrific," Keith said. "Let's do it." Becky saw her husband's hands reaching for her and jumped backward. Squealing and giggling, Becky squirmed away from Keith's extended fingers, resisting the inevitable one last time.

As she moved, Becky felt her foot slip between the mattress and the bed's ornate footboard. She tried to reach out to steady herself, but she clutched only air. She squealed again as she fell, thinking that after all the sexy stripping, she was going to ruin the mood with a stupid, awkward fall.

Keith reached for her and suddenly saw where she was going to land. As if in slow motion, he saw her legs straddle the slender bedpost and watched the candle-shaped wooden rod penetrate Becky's vagina.

The phone rang at about 12:45 in the morning. Because I was on duty that night, I came instantly awake. "Joan," the voice said, "I've got a hysterical man on the phone. All I can get out of him is that his wife's bleeding. The address is 227 Poppy. That's in the new Floral Court development."

"I know where it is," I answered. "Who else is on duty with me?"

"I've only got you and Sam Middleton," the police dispatcher said.

As I talked, I braced the phone between my shoulder and my ear and began to pull on my underwear. "Okay. Sam's closer to headquarters, so ask him to get the rig. Then set off the pagers and get at least one more person to the scene."

"Will do," the dispatcher said. "I've also got two of my units en route to the scene."

"Great." I hung up, finished dressing, and was out of my condo in less than 90 seconds.

Floral Court was only about two miles from my house, and I made it there quickly. As I turned onto Floral Way, the main road into the development, I started to peer at the street signs. "Rose Court, Daisy Drive." Thank God the development is so new that the street signs hadn't been torn up or turned by the local teenagers.

"Poppy." I made the left and saw the flashing lights of two police cars, already at the scene. I pulled up, grabbed the crash kit from my trunk, and ran into the house. "Hello," I called. "Ambulance."

"Up here." I recognized Chuck Harding's voice. I sprinted up the stairs and down the hall. The sight that greeted me was one that I will never forget.

The two officers, Chuck Harding and Will McAndrews, were standing just inside the bedroom staring at an unbelievable tableau. A naked woman was balanced on the end of the bed's footboard, supporting herself with her feet on the bed and frame and held around the waist by a bewildered-looking man I assumed to be her husband. Her loud moans filled the room. As I looked more carefully, I could see blood trickling down the wooden dowel, making a widening red stain on the gray carpeting. My mind went blank. I had no idea what to do.

In our training, we're taught some basic questions to ask when first evaluating a situation and taking a medical history. The first question, of course, is "What happened?" followed by, "What hurts?" All I could think of at that moment were those two questions and AMPLE, our acronym, which stands for Allergies, Medications, Past medical history, Last meal, and Events leading up to this occurrence. All I could do at that moment was fall back on those basic questions.

"What happened?"

"She fell," the man supporting the woman's body said. The woman moaned.

I walked slowly across the room and supported the woman on the side opposite her husband. "Ma'am," I said, "can you tell me what hurts?"

"That's a damn stupid question," the man said. "She's got a fuckin' bedpost rammed up her cunt and you ask what hurts."

That got my mind functioning. I was mad, but I had to admit that he was right. It was a dumb question. I had to do something, and do it fast. The woman was losing a considerable amount of blood. "Okay, sir, just relax."

"I'm sorry," he said. "I'm just so scared."

Now that my brain was working again, I realized what we had. An impaled object. "Never remove an impaled object," I remember my EMT instructor saying. "You never know what's being held together by the knife, or ice pick, or whatever." Or bedpost, I thought.

I turned to Chuck Harding. "Chuck, get the fire department's rescue truck out here. We'll need a saw or something to cut this bed apart. And see who is responding from FVAC."

"Cut the bed apart?" the man snapped. "You're out of your fuckin' mind. Just help me get her down from here. I can't lift her by myself."

"No, sir, we can't do that. We need to leave the post right there. It may be controlling a lot of bleeding. Just try to help us. What's your name?"

"Keith. I'm her husband."

"And hers?" I asked, indicating the moaning woman.

"Becky."

"Okay." I turned my attention to the woman. "Becky, we're going to get you down from there as soon as we can."

"Oh, god, it hurts so much." She began to cry.

"Becky, you have to stay as calm as you can. Please don't cry. It's important that you move as little as possible." She took a shuddering breath and stopped sobbing.

I heard Sam Middleton run into the bedroom, carrying the megaduffel. "Oh, shit," he said, staring at the woman impaled on the bedpost. "What can I do, Joan?"

"Come over here and help support her," I said. "Keith, let Sam take her weight. You get a blanket so we can cover her and keep her warm."

Thankful for something to do, Keith carefully surrendered Becky's care to Sam and me and pulled a granny-square afghan from the chair in the corner.

"Sam, we have to keep her still and I need to consult with the fire department about how we're going to get her down." As crew chief, it was my job to coordinate rescue operations. I looked at the remaining police officer. "Will, can you take over from me?"

Will McAndrews walked over and stood next to me. "Tell me what to do," he said.

"It's most important that she not move. Any change in position might do more internal damage. Lift her by her underarm and take her weight from me." As Will took over from me, I said to the woman, "Becky, I know it hurts, but just be patient a little longer and try not to move."

"I'll try," she whispered.

As I was freed from holding Becky, I heard Phil Ortiz's voice from behind me. "Holy shit," he said, then looked embarrassed and slammed his mouth shut. Phil was a good EMT and a new riding member, but he was only eighteen. "Phil," I said, "set me up a non-rebreather on twelve liters." Phil hesitated, staring at the tableau before him. "NOW, Phil," I said, bringing him out of his reverie. He slowly reached for the megaduffel and pulled out the oxygen equipment.

While Phil was working, I wondered what else I could do for Becky. I ticked off the treatments for severe bleeding. Direct pressure; not for internal injuries. Elevate the injury site; we obviously couldn't do that either. Treat for shock by administering high-flow oxygen; Phil was taking care of that. Maintain body temperature. I felt the skin on the woman's leg. Her flesh was cold. "Keith," I said, "get me another blanket and then turn the heat in the house up as far as it will go."

Happy to again be able to help, Keith got a blanket from the closet, then disappeared down the stairs. Phil handed me an oxygen mask, attached to an O_2 cylinder. As I placed the mask over Becky's face, I said, "This will help you. Just breathe normally." I turned to Phil, who still appeared distracted. "Hand me a BP cuff and stethoscope."

Phil seemed not to hear me and kept staring at the bleeding patient. I pulled him out into the hall. "Phil, you've got to try to pull yourself together. We need you."

"But she's . . ."

I spoke to him calmly. "She's going to be in worse shape if we can't help her. You're going to have to make a very quick decision. Either you're part of this crew or I'll have the police page out for more manpower." I hoped that there were more people responding anyway, but I had to get Phil to begin to function, as much for himself as for our patient. We've lost several good EMTs after bad calls like this. They face the helplessness and frustration and begin to doubt themselves. I wanted Phil to know, as I did, that he could handle himself in a crisis.

Phil took a deep breath and nodded. "I'm with you. It's just so horrible."

I put my arm around his shoulders. "I know, but we have to do the best we can for her. We can both fall apart later, if we need to. And we've worked together enough that I know you can handle this."

Phil nodded again. "BP cuff and stethoscope coming up." Together, we walked back into the room. Phil went directly over to the megaduffel and unzipped the end compartment, retrieved the equipment to take vitals, and handed it to me. "I'll take care of the PCR," Phil said.

Keith and Chuck Harding returned together. "Heat's all the way up," Keith said, then returned to his wife.

"Fire Rescue is rolling," the officer said, "and 45–22 is en route." I was never so happy to learn that Ed was responding. I considered contacting the helicopter, then quickly discarded the idea. At that time it responded only from 7

A.M. to 7 P.M. We had been promised 24-hour service, but it hadn't started yet.

While Phil began to gather information for our PCR, I took Becky's vitals. "Phil," I said when I was done, "BP one hundred ten over seventy-six, pulse one hundred, respirations about thirty and shallow." Her vitals showed that so far her body was coping adequately with the blood loss. How long that would continue, I didn't know.

While Phil entered the information on the report, I tried to keep Becky calm. "Are you warm enough?" I asked her.

"I guess. How long?"

At that moment I heard another siren. "I think that's the rescue truck now," I said, hoping I was right. "They'll have you down in just a few moments." I'm going to go downstairs and fill them in. Sam, that's my EMT friend here, and Will—he's the fuzz, so don't say anything incriminating—will stay with you." I realize that I say some of the most inane things under stress sometimes, but I want so desperately to calm my patient.

Becky looked at me and gave a tiny smile. "Just hurry."

"I'm here, too, honey," Keith said. "Hang on to me." He reached out and took Becky's hand.

I hurried down the stairs and out the front door and saw the fire department rescue truck parked at the curb. A dozen burly firefighters in full turnout gear milled around the lawn. I looked for the person in the white helmet and spotted Chief Palmer. "Chief," I called. "We need to talk, quick."

"What's the situation?"

I saw Ed get out of his car, and I waved him over. Using as few words as possible, I explained the situation to both of them.

"Unless we can take the footboard apart," Chief Palmer said, "we'll have to cut through the post." I could see his mind working. Both the Fairfax Police Department and the Fairfax Volunteer Fire Department are staffed by some of the most helpful and cooperative people I've ever met.

They understand what we do and they're always ready with support and suggestions.

"If the post is too long," Ed said, "the victim won't fit into the rig."

"True," I said. "And Chief, whatever we do, let's try to keep the number of people in the bedroom down to a minimum."

The chief selected two of his men while Ed got a backboard from the rig. Ed carried the board, and together with the three firefighters, one with a full toolbox in hand, we went back into the house.

When we reentered the bedroom, the scene was unchanged. Quickly, the three firemen assessed the situation and examined the bed. "This footboard and the bedposts, it's all one piece. It won't come apart," one firefighter said softly.

The chief nodded, then turned to me. "We're going to have to saw through the post right here." He showed me a narrow spot, just above where the post joined the footboard. "What do you think, Grant," the chief asked the firefighter who had examined the wood, "handsaw?"

"Won't touch this wood," he answered. "How about the power saw?"

The chief considered. "Too much vibration. Let's try the jaws."

"Sounds like the best alternative," the one called Grant said.

While the three of them went back outside to connect the cutting attachment to the jaws of life, I tried to reassure the husband and wife. "I know you hurt, Becky, but it will be only a little while longer." I looked at Chuck and Sam, still supporting the woman. "Are you two okay for now? Do you want Ed or Phil to relieve you?"

"We're fine for now," Sam said.

The three firemen returned, dragging the cutting tool, attached by pneumatic hoses to the generator downstairs. Phil ran to get the stretcher while I changed places with Sam. He and Ed raised the longboard behind the weakening woman and used it to support her back. Two firefighters held the post and another wielded the cutting tool. The jaws made quick work of the wood, and soon Becky was being pressed against the backboard and lowered to the stretcher, the remains of the post still extending from between her legs.

We used the upper sheet from the stretcher and several large safety pins to bind Becky's legs together and stabilize the post. We then strapped her, longboard and all, to the stretcher and started toward St. Luke's. Despite the fact that Sam drove at only 20 miles per hour in some places, and avoided as many bumps as he could, every movement of the rig caused Becky to scream. While I held her head, Phil took her hand. Somehow, he had come to terms with his initial hesitation.

We arrived at the hospital in about 12 minutes and rushed Becky into the ER. Before we finished our cleanup, she was on her way upstairs, first to X-ray, then to the operating room. Dr. Englander, the trauma specialist on duty, walked over and said, "Nice work, guys. One false move and she would have bled to death while you watched. Any idea how she got herself into that predicament?"

"I don't think I want to speculate," I answered.

"What are her chances?" Phil asked.

"Pretty good," the doctor said. "Her vitals weren't too bad and, if the X-rays don't show more internal damage than I think they will, she'll be okay. I don't know about her ever having children, though. That'll be up to the surgeon and what he sees when he opens her up."

"God," Phil said, his eyes wide, "I hope she'll be all right."

The doctor put his arm around Phil's shoulders and said, "Feel free to call tomorrow or the next day and we'll let you know."

The following day, I got a call from Phil. "She'll be okay," he said joyously. "I called ICU. She'll be pretty bad for a little while, but they're reasonably sure that she's going to make it. The nurse said that eventually she'll be good as new. In every way."

"That's great. And how about you? Are you okay? We can get someone from the crisis debriefing team to talk to you, you know."

"I know and I've gotten lectured from both the captain and my mother. But I'm okay, really."

"That's great. And by the way, despite what you might be thinking, you were fine on that call."

"Do you think so? I froze. I just couldn't function at all. I don't know what I'd have done if you hadn't given me that pep talk."

"Everyone has bad moments, now and then. I must admit that when I first saw the situation, my mind went blank, too. We all freeze, or we make a mistake. Accept that we're all human and all we can do is the best that we can do. We're not superhuman, although often we'd like to be."

"You froze, too? Last night?"

"For a few moments I had no idea what to do and I was the only EMT. So I fell back on the basics and did *something*. When I came down from my own sort of autopilot I discovered that I hadn't done any harm. So just be sure to get help if you need it, and move on. But don't give up. The ones that we feel good about far outnumber the ones that go badly."

"I know. And I'll be fine."

"I'm sure you will. See you soon."

"Yup. See ya."

The most wonderful experience I've had as an EMT began early one icy morning in January. Ed had just left my house to go to work when the pagers went off.

"Fairfax Police to all home units. One additional crew member is needed on Route 10 near Route 541 for a woman in labor. Any available units, please call in."

Normally a call for a woman in labor is just a transport. Because of good prenatal care and education, mothers-to-be usually have enough warning to get to the hospital in good time. I have had plenty of those transports, but I wanted to go just in case. I called the police and told them I would respond directly to the scene, just a few blocks from my condo.

"312 to anyone responding to the call for the woman in labor. Be extremely careful," I heard the police officer say as I dressed. "The roads are very icy."

I heard Steve Nesbitt answer from FVAC headquarters. "10–4. I just arrived and it's terrible out there. Be advised," he continued, "the ETA for the rig is at least ten minutes." Because it was already 8:15 and I know that Steve drives a school bus, I assumed that the schools were all closed because of the ice.

I ran out of my apartment and was immediately pelted with a miserable mixture of rain and ice. As my foot touched the front walk, it slid out from under me and I landed on my hip. I stood up and slowly made my way to my car, rubbing my sore side. I scraped half an inch of hard ice off my windshield thinking, *Oh shit. If I'm going to arrive safely, I'll have to drive at a crawl.*

I reached Route 541 about five minutes later and saw a 1985 Chevy resting at a crazy angle off the side of the road in front of Fairfax Police car 312. I parked and skated across the roadway to the passenger side of the car.

An obviously pregnant woman sat in the passenger seat, grimacing. Sweat was running down the sides of her face despite the freezing weather. A man whom I took to be her husband was bending over her. Will McAndrews was standing next to the car looking helpless.

"My name is Joan," I said to anyone who was listening, "and I'm with the Ambulance Corps. What happened?"

The man looked up. "We were driving toward Fairfax Hospital because my wife is in labor. I couldn't keep the car on the road, and it just slid off the edge into this ditch. I couldn't get it out, so I flagged down this cop and he called for the ambulance."

"Was anyone injured?" I asked him.

"No. We slid off the side of the road very slowly. My wife wasn't even jostled, thank God."

As I watched, the woman's face began to relax. "Was that a contraction?" I asked.

"A beauty."

"What's your name?"

"Brenda. Brenda Bergman. And I'm having a baby." I smiled at her and, slightly embarrassed, she said, "I guess that's pretty obvious."

"I guess so," I said. The question was how soon. "How long have you been in labor?"

"I've been in labor about four hours." Four hours, I thought. No hurry. Labor usually lasts from 12 to 20 hours.

"How bad are the contractions?"

Her next words made me think again about how much time we had. "For the last half an hour I've been having push pains."

The front of her jumpsuit was soaked. "I gather your water has broken."

"About an hour ago." Her face began to contort again and she started to breathe in short, panting breaths.

"Another contraction?" I asked.

Brenda nodded and I looked at my watch. "They're about a minute and a half apart," I said. "Is that about right?" I swallowed hard. A minute and a half. Holy cow.

She nodded again. Icy rain-sleet was running down my neck as I turned to her husband. "Is this her first baby?" I asked. First children come more slowly.

"It's our second. The last time, she was in labor only four hours," he answered.

Oh, shit, I thought. Not much time at all. I was delighted about the possible opportunity to deliver a baby but suddenly scared by the responsibility.

I heard a siren, glanced up, and said, "Here's the ambulance, Brenda. Soon we'll be able to make you more comfortable."

The ambulance pulled up and I saw Ed get out. "How did you get here?" I asked.

"I decided to stop at headquarters on my way home to find out whether there was a full crew on duty. I had just walked into the garage when the call came in."

"I think we may have to deliver this one," I said.

Ed and Steve brought the stretcher up next to the car and held a yellow plastic sheet over the car door to try to keep Brenda dry.

"Brenda," I said, "as you get onto the stretcher, I want you to slip out of your slacks and your underwear so I can examine you."

"Do you think you're going to have to deliver the baby in the ambulance?" Brenda asked.

"I'd love to deliver a baby," Ed said as Brenda undressed. "What a thrill. Unfortunately, though, the trip to FGH should take only ten minutes. Unless the baby's crowning now, it'll probably wait until we get to the hospital."

"I'll examine you when we get into the rig," I said as we lifted Brenda into the ambulance. I asked her husband to join us in the rig, but he said that he had to wait for the tow truck and would meet his wife in the labor room.

Ed and I climbed into the back of the rig and Steve got into the driver's seat.

I examined Brenda while Ed took vitals. "I don't see any evidence of the baby's head, Brenda," I said, replacing the sheet and blanket over her legs and abdomen. "I think that the baby will wait until we get to Fairfax General." Ed nodded. Brenda's vitals were fine.

"Okay, Steve, let's go, but take it slow and easy. We're fine back here."

Brenda panted through another contraction, but even at its peak, the baby's head was still not visible. As the rig made its slow progress toward the hospital, Brenda, Ed, and I talked.

"Maple's blocked with a three-car accident, Joan," Steve called from the front. "I'm going to turn around and go back along Route 10 to Mill Street. I may use the parkway. It will probably be the first thing sanded."

"Are we going to be very long?" Brenda asked.

"You heard Steve," I said. "We'll do what we have to do, and Steve's the best. He drives a school bus for a living and he knows the town like the back of his hand. There are several alternate routes we can take to the hospital and I'm sure that not all of them are blocked. And if the baby decides to be born in the ambulance, we'll handle that, too."

"Have you ever delivered a baby?" Brenda asked.

"No, neither Ed nor I have. But we have been well trained in childbirth procedures and we know how to take the best care of both you and your baby. Anyway, doctors don't deliver babies, they just catch them. Mothers do all the work and you've had some practice." I hoped I sounded confident. I was confident of our ability to handle the birth if everything went normally. Yet part of me was thinking of all the things that could go wrong.

"We've got a sander in front of us, sanding our way to the hospital," Steve called. "We should be there in about ten minutes."

"That's good," Brenda said. "I'm sure you can do whatever is necessary, but I'd rather my doctor handle the delivery."

We filled out the prehospital care report and talked for about five minutes, interrupted by more contractions, and then felt the rig stop. "What now?"

"We were doing fine until the sander in front of us got stuck," Steve yelled from the front. "Looks like we're here for a while. Traffic's backed up solid in both directions."

I looked at Brenda and shrugged. As I looked out the back window of the rig I saw that Steve was right—we were there for the duration.

"Why don't you come in the back with us, Steve?" Ed said through the window that connects the cab with the box on the back, "at least until they get that sander going. Maybe we'll have the great honor of delivering a baby after all."

Brenda was just starting to pant, and I leaned over and removed the sheet and blanket covering her lower body. At the peak of the contraction, I saw her tissues part and the top of a head begin to appear. "Well, Brenda, it looks like your baby is going to be born right here."

Ed and I opened the OB kit, and as Ed spread out all the equipment we would need, I pulled on a pair of sterile gloves. Steve climbed into the back of the rig, and I suggested that he sit by Brenda's head and be responsible for psychological first aid for her. Ed would take care of the baby. I would take care of Brenda.

"How are you doing, Brenda? Contractions worse?"

"The pains are about as bad as they get," Brenda said. "Will we be okay?"

"We'll be fine," I said, hoping I was right.

With the next contraction I saw the baby's head emerge through the mass of amniotic fluid and blood. I positioned my hands as I had been taught and pressed my palm lightly against the tiny head to prevent the baby from emerging too fast.

Despite the slight pressure, as the next contraction began, I was amazed at how quickly the baby began to slip out. I slid my hand under the baby's shoulders and wrapped my fingers around a tiny arm. Both ankles emerged and I grabbed them with the other hand as I remembered the nurse doing in the movie I had seen in EMT class. I remember thinking that she had been right about another fact. Babies are amazingly slippery.

So much could still go wrong, I thought as I prayed for the baby to begin breathing. I held the newborn with its head lower than its body while Ed suctioned fluid out of its mouth and nose. As if on cue, the baby caught a breath and began to wail.

Everyone in the ambulance began to laugh. I handed the baby to Ed and took sterile towels and pads and began to clean Brenda up. Ed wiped the tiny face and quickly wrapped the baby in a receiving blanket and put it on Brenda's stomach. Brenda reached down and touched the baby's fingers.

"It's so beautiful," I said. It. All at once, we realized that none of us had checked the baby's sex. Ed unwrapped the blanket and grinned. "Brenda, you have a son. What's his name?"

"His name is David. I can't decide whether to laugh or cry. He's so wonderful."

"Ed," I said, "why don't you call the hospital on the radio and let them know that David Bergman, born at," I glanced at my watch, "9:12 A.M., is healthy and wonderful, as is his mom. The hospital should be able to get word to Mr. Bergman, too."

After Ed finished the radio message, we talked and laughed and cried. The baby cried for a while and finally managed to put his fist in his mouth. After about 15 minutes, we heard a knock on the side door. Steve opened it, and a gruff voice said, "We'll be able to get you folks goin' in about a minute. Everyone okay?"

"We're terrific," I said. "Just terrific."

It was another 20 minutes before the rig pulled into the emergency entrance of Fairfax General. As Ed opened the back doors, we all saw a large group of nurses, doctors, and people in civilian clothes, applauding. We quickly wheeled mother and baby up to the maternity floor where Brenda's doctor was waiting.

"You did good work," the doctor said as he examined Brenda. "She looks fine and so does the baby."

"Don't you think the crew is entitled to part of your fee, Doctor?" I asked.

He grinned. "Send me a bill, and I'll consider it."

○ ○ ○

NEIL WALSH'S FIRST name wasn't really Neil. It was Edgar. As a child, he had always hated Edgar and now he had almost forgotten his real name. In high school, he had taken the name of his idol, Neil Diamond, and the name stuck.

Neil was a soft-spoken man of twenty-eight, married, with two small children when Jim and Wendy Frankel moved in next door with their three children. The two couples became immediate friends. Jim had a long-standing interest in hunting and, although Neil couldn't abide guns, he learned to tolerate Jim's favorite sport, bow-hunting. Once or twice a season he'd let Jim take him to some wooded location and he'd sit in the fresh air with a cross-bow, aiming at nothing.

It was a particularly cold morning, mid-winter, 1986, as Neil and Jim trudged across the familiar snow-covered electric company right-of-way near Fairfax. Neil had put on two sets of thermal underwear, a sweater, and a one-piece flannel coverall. His final layer was a heavyweight camouflage jumpsuit. Wearing three pairs of socks, heavy work boots, and two woolen caps, he was warm and comfortable even though the temperature hovered around 15 degrees.

"What a fantastic morning," Neil said, enjoying the cold sunlight. He took a deep breath. "But it freezes my nose."

"Let's split up," Jim said. He motioned toward a wooden platform anchored to a tree about ten feet off the ground. "You take your favorite spot over there, and I'll head off that way. I'll meet you at the car in," he dug under his gloves and sleeve and checked his watch, "three hours." Jim plodded off through the three or four inches of snow and over the crest of a small rise.

Neil boosted himself up onto the platform and settled into a comfortable position. Long before, he had decided that he wasn't interested in actually shooting anything so, as usual, he settled back and let his mind wander. About an hour later he pulled a chocolate bar from the pocket of his jumpsuit and ate a few bites.

Suddenly, some of the chocolate tickled his throat and he started to cough. The sound of his coughing covered the sound of cracking wood.

"Fairfax Police to Fairfax Ambulance."

"Go ahead Fairfax Police."

"The ambulance is needed behind 3772 Spring Hill Street for someone who has fallen in the woods."

"Ten-four. 45–01 is responding."

I was a new probationary member, taking my first EMT course, so I climbed into the back of the rig and tried to figure out what we were in for this time. "Don't look so tense, Joan," Linda Potemski said, as if she could read my mind. "Bob's crew chief. All you have to do is follow instructions. You'll do fine." She was right. I wouldn't have to initiate any action, only take direction from Linda and the senior crew members, Jack McCaffrey and Bob Fiorella.

When the rig arrived at the driveway on Spring Hill, we saw the police waving us toward a wooded area behind the house. Six inches of snow had fallen three days before, and because only the shadowy areas were still snow-covered, I was wearing only sneakers. As we trudged through the snow, I was concentrating on the lump of fabric toward whom two Fairfax policemen were leading us. There, lying half-propped against a hollow tree trunk, we found a man in his mid-twenties dressed in a one-piece fatigue jumpsuit. Jack placed one hand on each side of the man's head.

Bob, who was officially crew chief that afternoon, put down the crash bag, leaned over, and looked the man in the eye. "What happened?" Although apparently conscious, the man said nothing. Bob turned to Will McAndrews, the police officer who had been first on the scene.

"He seems to have fallen from this blind," the policeman said, pointing to a hunting platform in the tree about ten feet above the ground. "From what I can gather from his friend," the policeman said, motioning toward another fatigue-clad man standing a few feet to one side, "the two men separated about ten this morning to hunt deer. They agreed to meet a couple of hours later. When Neil here," he pointed to our patient, "didn't show up, his friend went looking, finally found him here and called us."

I looked up at the platform and saw that the side and part of the floor were broken. A crossbow and a scattering of arrows lay in the snow beside Neil.

"Neil," Bob said loudly, "can you hear me?" Neil's eyes moved and we knew he was dimly aware of our presence, but his level of consciousness was severely depressed.

"Jack," Bob said, controlling the situation, "maintain head stabilization and don't move." He turned to me. "Joan, you and Linda get the Reeves and the collar bag." I visualized the slatted stretcher that would wrap around Neil so we could carry him through the woods.

"No longboard?" Linda asked. "It is better support for his neck and back."

"I'd love to use a longboard," Bob continued, half to himself, "but we'd have trouble getting him through this scrub. And you'd better bring some blankets, too. This guy is severely hypothermic."

From his position behind Neil's head, Jack said, "Maybe you'd better bring the rig as close as you can, but don't drive off the pavement. The bouncing getting out will play hell with the patient."

"Good idea," Bob said. This type of interchange was why I loved working with this crew. No egos, just four people trying to do the best for their patients. On other crews, the crew chief was considered God and no one argued with the way he wanted to handle the situation.

Linda and I trudged back through the snow to the ambulance. Now that my initial adrenaline rush was beginning to wear off, I was becoming aware of my feet. They were starting to feel like blocks of ice. I thought about warming them in the rig for a moment, but I realized that although I wanted to stay in the warm ambulance, I had a job to do.

I walked behind the rig while Linda turned it around and backed it as far down the long driveway as she could. Then we assembled three blankets, the collar bag, and the Reeves stretcher and carried them back to Neil. Although each time I crossed the snowy areas I tried to walk in existing footsteps, my shoes were full of snow and my toes were becoming numb. I silently vowed that from October to March, I would always have boots handy when on duty.

By the time we returned to the tree, Bob had freed one of our patient's arms from his fatigues and had gotten a first set of vitals. "All his vitals are depressed. Pulse is only forty-four, respiration's ten. BP is one hundred over seventy." We wanted to say more about Neil's serious condition, but we couldn't talk freely where he might be listening. Bob and Jack began to maneuver Neil's clothes out of the way so they could get the cervical collar around his neck.

"Can we take his temperature so we know how cold he is?" I asked Linda.

"Our thermometers won't register below about ninety-four degrees. This guy's probably down into the eighties."

"How do you know that?" I asked.

"When the core temperature falls below about ninety degrees, the body stops shivering." She pointed to Neil. "He's not shivering and probably hasn't been for a while. Now we have to figure out how to move him with the least additional damage."

I looked at the position Neil was in and at the tree, and I was glad that I didn't have to make any decisions as to how to get him onto the Reeves. I had no idea how Bob would accomplish it without compromising his neck and spine.

"This won't be easy," Bob said. "Joan, change places with Jack. You be in charge of Neil's head and take special care to support his neck and spine. Jack, I need your muscle down here."

I looked at where Jack was standing and realized that I would have to climb through a snowdrift and into the hollow of the tree to take over from him. I tried to stay as dry as I could as I scrambled into the tree and gently, without any movement, took over head stabilization.

Standing inside the tree in a bed of leaves and damp debris, I supported Neil's head while Bob, Linda, and Jack fastened the extrication collar around his neck. Positioning themselves, they prepared to pull him down flat, then log-roll him onto the Reeves.

"It's almost over now, Neil," I said, not knowing whether he could hear me. "We'll have you out of here and into a warm ambulance in just a few minutes."

"Let's get ready to roll him," Bob said as he gave everyone a specific task, straightening and arranging Neil's limbs and setting up the Reeves. I had the easiest task. I would just turn and support his head as we rolled. But my job was the most critical as well. One false move and any broken vertebrae might do additional damage to Neil's fragile spinal cord. Because I was at the head, I would also control the timing of the move.

When we were all ready, Bob said, "On your count, Joan."

Softly, I said to Neil, "We're going to move you now. Try to relax and let us do all the work." I looked at the crew and said, "One, two, three." We straightened Neil's limbs and turned his torso, then Bob used his free hand to push the folded stretcher snugly against Neil's back. Throughout the procedure, which must have caused him some pain, Neil was silent, his face composed, his limbs flaccid.

When everyone was ready, I said, "Now back. One, two, three." Neil was finally on the stretcher, his body, head, and neck padded with blankets. We rolled the Reeves as tightly around him as we could, then, while I carried equipment and continued to talk to him, Bob, Linda, Jack, and the policeman each took a corner of the Reeves and carried Neil back through the woods to the ambulance.

In the rig, we peeled open Neil's fatigue jumpsuit and his second layer. When we cut through a soft light-blue sweater and two layers of thermal underwear I could feel his cold skin. We cranked the heat in the back of the rig as high as we could and put a non-rebreather oxygen mask on him. With Jack driving, we started toward the medical center, lights and siren.

Bob checked for pain responses in Neil's hands. "No response," Bob muttered.

Linda reached over. "Let me try a sternal rub." She pressed a knuckle against Neil's breastbone and twisted. I looked at Neil's face as I imagined the sudden pain that should have caused. Neil's face remained impassive.

I leaned toward Bob and, over the wail of the siren, I asked quietly, "Can hypothermia cause this?"

Bob answered, facing away from Neil so he couldn't hear, "I suspect that he's not just hypothermic. I think he's got a broken neck and he's got no feeling from the neck down."

Suddenly his relaxation during our logroll made sense. Oh, God, I thought. Paralyzed. One moment healthy, hunting deer with a bow and arrow. The next, this.

We pulled into the ambulance parking area of the medical center and unloaded our patient. Bob finished the paperwork, and we left, without knowing much about his condition. The next morning the newspaper confirmed what Bob had feared. Edgar (Neil) Walsh had three broken vertebrae and was paralyzed from the neck down.

In the years since, there have been several articles in our local paper about Neil's progress. The most recent one says that he's regained some use of his arms. He still vows that he will walk again.

ALPHABET SOUP

AS WITH ANY other professional group, EMS, the emergency medical services, has its own language and its own abbreviations. Below are some of the ones more frequently used.

ASAP—As Soon As Possible
BP—Blood Pressure
BVM—Bag Valve Mask—a device that forces air or pure oxygen into a patient's lungs. It can be used during CPR or to assist inadequate respirations.
CCU—Cardiac Care Unit—area in a hospital specially equipped to care for victims of heart attacks.
CPR—Cardio-Pulmonary Resuscitation—the process of using external means to circulate the blood or fill the lungs with oxygen or both.
EDP—Emotionally Disturbed Person
EKG—electrocardiogram—a tracing that indicates the electrical activity within the heart's muscle and nervous system.
EMD—Electrical Mechanical Dissociation—a condition in which electrical impulses exist in a heart, but they are unable to stimulate normal contractions.
EMT—Emergency Medical Technician
EMT-D—an EMT with added training in defibrillation, jump starting a stopped heart with a controlled electrical shock. Most of the EMTs in FVAC are EMT-Ds.
ER—Emergency Room

ETA—Estimated Time of Arrival

FGH—Fairfax General Hospital, the smaller, community hospital that serves the fictional town of Fairfax. In addition to this hospital, down the parkway there is a county medical facility and trauma center.

FVAC—abbreviation for the fictional Fairfax Volunteer Ambulance Corps. It is pronounced eff vac.

ICU—Intensive Care Unit—area in a hospital specially equipped to care for people in serious condition.

IV—Intravenous

KED—Kendrick Extrication Device—a brand-name product. The KED is a plastic-covered, vertically slatted jacket used to immobilize the head, neck, and spine of a victim of an accident in order to minimize additional trauma while he is being moved.

MAST—Military Anti-Shock Trousers—pants with inflatable bladders in each leg and the abdomen that can be pressurized like a BP cuff. Inflation usually slows the deterioration of a patient in shock. PASG, pneumatic anti-shock garment, is another acronym for the same piece of apparatus.

MCI—Multiple Casualty Incident

MVA—Motor Vehicle Accident

OR—Operating Room

PCR—Prehospital Care Report—The report that our state requires us to fill in for every call we take.

PDAA—Property Damage Auto Accident

PIAA—Personal Injury Auto Accident

PFA—Psychological First Aid

RMA—Refused Medical Attention—a patient always has the right to refuse to let us care for him. It is, of course, our job to try to convince an ill or injured person to let us help him, but sometimes all our persuasion fails.

TLC—Tender Loving Care

NINE

IT SEEMS SO clear in the EMT class. We are taught neat and specific procedures for every emergency. All we have to do is learn them. Right?

Wrong!

A case in point are the procedures on how to deal with gunshot wounds.

To realize how unusual gunshot wounds are in a quiet suburban town like Fairfax, you must know that the corps has had only five or six calls for shootings in the 15 years that I've been a member. I've had to deal with two of them. I remember each call with amazing clarity, the first almost eight years ago, the second only about a year ago.

Stan Poritsky noticed a man sitting in the darkened car as he drove into the local park on his regular patrol. It had been a quiet shift: a couple of burglar alarms—both false as usual, a barking dog complaint, three routine traffic stops. As he drove through the greenery and past the still-busy tennis court, he saw nothing out of the ordinary: a man walking a dog, a woman out late jogging, a few pairs of teens necking on the grass.

As he neared the park exit, Officer Poritsky stopped his car for a few moments to do some paperwork. Although it was quiet, he somehow didn't hear the gunshot in the car just a few feet away.

He finished his writing and returned to the entrance. On his way out he noticed that the man was now slumped over the steering wheel.

Drunk or sleeping, he thought. *Probably had a fight with his wife and needed to get away.*

Stan pulled up alongside the parked car, got out of his police cruiser, and looked in at the slumped figure. He shined his flashlight into the car and he saw the blood splattered over the man's face and the front of his white sweatshirt. As the officer opened the driver's side door, he spotted the handgun dangling from the man's limp fingers.

At FVAC headquarters we could hear the shock and panic in his voice as the cop radioed his headquarters. "Get the ambulance to the main park entrance, ASAP. I've got a man with a gunshot wound."

Jack McCaffrey jumped from his chair and keyed the mike. "FVAC to PD. We read your officer direct and are responding."

I remember the fear that I felt as we sped toward the scene. Who did the shooting? Is he still there? Is there more than one victim by now? We all knew that our first priority on any call is our own safety, but because there was an officer already there, the scene should be safe. Should be . . .

We pulled up, and Officer Poritsky ran over to us. "Self-inflicted gunshot wound to the head. There's so much blood, but I think he's still alive."

We ran over to the car and Stan shined his light into the passenger compartment. I looked in through the passenger-side window and saw the blood. It was unlike anything I had encountered before. I recall my feeling of utter helplessness in the face of the massive trauma of a gunshot wound to the head. As Jack checked the man, it became obvious to all of us that the wound was probably fatal. The amount of blood and tissue splashed around the passenger compartment was not compatible with life.

"He's still got a pulse," Jack said, "and he's breathing."

We all responded instinctively. We didn't even consider all the specific procedures for dealing with trauma: Direct pressure, elevation, treat for shock. We just "scooped and ran," barely taking time to apply several multitrauma dressings to his head and to hold them in place with three rolls of Kling bandages. We slid the man's body onto a longboard and loaded him into the rig. On the way to St. Luke's Trauma Center, we put him on oxygen, checked his weak vitals, put on and inflated the MAST.

He was still alive when we reached the hospital, but we all knew that everyone was just going through the motions. No one could survive such a massive head wound. There was nothing we could have done.

It was years later when the tones went off and an excited police dispatcher said, "The rig is needed in front of 401 Main for a man with a gunshot wound to the chest. Officer requests you expedite."

Because we have so few calls like this, I flashed back eight years to the man in the car. I was crew chief this time and as we sped to the scene, I reviewed everything I knew about gunshot wounds. Scene safety first. A bullet hole in the chest would probably produce a sucking chest wound, one that would allow air to enter the lung cavity and prevent adequate breathing. I would have to seal the hole to aid his breathing. I would also have to remember to look for an exit wound.

As we approached the scene, I saw three police cars already on location. Multicolored strobe lights splashed the darkened area with bizarre colors. *Okay, at least we're safe,* I thought. No gunman waiting to shoot us, too.

Two officers I didn't immediately recognize were trying to control about a dozen curious bystanders who surrounded someone on the ground. "Come on, folks. Let the ambulance crew through," one of them said.

We pulled the stretcher and a longboard from the rig. I had no idea yet what we'd need, so I yelled to Steve Nesbitt, "Get the duffel and bring the suction."

The scene was bedlam. "Help him!" somebody screamed.

"I can't believe it!"

"He's dead, he's dead!"

"He killed himself."

One woman merely repeated, "He was such a nice man. He always seemed like such a nice man," over and over.

As we approached, one of the cops yelled, "Get a stretcher over here and get him going fast."

We wheeled the stretcher toward the figure on the ground, but before I could say anything, three heavyset men picked the man up by his arms and legs and dumped him on the stretcher. "Help him! You gotta get him to the hospital!" one of them shrieked at us.

I looked at the man, his chest covered with blood. So much for careful handling. Whatever damage could be done by moving the man carelessly had already been done. One of the crew members put a non-rebreather oxygen mask on the patient's face and another helped me strap the man onto the stretcher. As we hustled to the rig, I noticed one of the cops holding a rifle covered with blood. As we lifted the victim into the ambulance, I wondered how a man could shoot himself in the chest with a rifle.

Inside, I said to the driver, "Give me a minute to examine him and get some vitals." One of the other crew members had already cut the man's shirt open and I could see and hear his chest wound. It didn't really make a sucking sound, as my training had predicted. It gurgled through the waves of flowing blood. *Seal the hole,* I thought. I reached down to place the palm of my gloved hand on the wound.

Suddenly the man started flailing his arms, trying to get off the stretcher. Despite the stretcher straps, he was twisting his body around, causing more blood to flow from his chest wound. My partner and I each grabbed a shoulder and held him down.

"Lie still!" I yelled at him. "We're trying to help you!" He was amazingly strong despite his massive wound and loss of blood, and he continued to fight us. "We'll have to restrain him," I said to Steve. It was a struggle, but between us we managed to tie his wrists to the sidebars of the stretcher.

"To hell with vitals. Let's move," I yelled to our driver, realizing that we had already spent much too much time at the scene. I would seal the chest wound as we rushed to the hospital. So much for checking for an exit wound.

While Steve sealed the wound with his hand, I grabbed the Saran Wrap, tore off a long sheet, folded it several times, and placed it over the wound. I remembered the illustration in my EMT textbook and tried to make the dressing look like the picture. Steve released his pressure, and I pressed the patch against the wound. "Tape the edges," I said.

Steve tore off a strip of tape and unsuccessfully tried to tape the edge of the plastic to the man's chest. "Shit," he said. "I can't make this stuff stick."

I now recalled that the picture in the EMT book had been of a neat wound on a dry, hairless chest. This man's chest was covered with hair and the hair was floating in blood.

"Try wider tape," I suggested, then I remembered that we had to leave one corner open. As the man inhaled, the plastic would seal the wound, allowing no air to enter the chest cavity through the chest wall, thus enabling him to breathe. As he exhaled, the seal would loosen and permit the pressure within the chest cavity to lessen. "And we need to leave a corner open," I said, then realized how ridiculous that sounded. We would be lucky if we got anything to stick. Finally, using the widest tape in the ambulance and wrapping it around to the man's back, we were able to keep the plastic in place over most of the wound.

We attempted to get vital signs and calm the man, but he continued to struggle. As I watched the needle on the blood pressure cuff drop, I suddenly became aware of a strong, pungent odor and saw that the side of the stretcher had become a waterfall of blood, blood that now flowed over the floor of the ambulance.

"Holy shit," I muttered. I had never seen so much blood appear so suddenly. I had never realized that blood had such a strong smell. "Steve . . ."

We stared at the chest wound, but that was not the source of all the blood. Steve pointed to a dark red river flowing over the side of the stretcher.

"Shit," he said, "it's coming from his back." It was gushing from the exit wound that we had never been able to look for. But, I realized, it wouldn't have made any difference. In his struggling, a major blood vessel must have let go. No dressing in the world would have helped.

By the time we reached the hospital our patient had stopped struggling. He died a few minutes after we got him into the ER.

○ ○ ○

I WAS AT the nurse's desk in the emergency room, writing up my prehospital care report on the forty-five-year-old man we had just brought in. He had been driving alone and, because he didn't remember what had happened, I assume that he had probably fallen asleep at the wheel. Fortunately, bushes had slowed his car before he hit the tree, so, although the car had been demolished, he remained relatively uninjured. Some cuts and bruises. Maybe a broken wrist.

That he had emerged in good shape from a totally wrecked car surprised me. Because the front and rear ends of today's cars are built to collapse upon impact, to absorb shock, and the passenger compartments are reinforced, people often emerge from bad front- or rear-end accidents with only minor injuries, provided that they are restrained by seat belts or, better still, by both seat belts and an air bag. But this man had simply beaten the odds. He had no air bag and had not been wearing a seat belt.

"What a lucky son of a bitch," I muttered to Rosemary Harper, the head nurse, who was sitting next to me, taking a coffee break. "He wasn't even wearing a seat belt."

"I never wear a seat belt," Rosemary replied, gulping the rancid brew produced by the ER coffee maker. The machine had not been cleaned for years, and even its freshly brewed coffee tasted like it had been on the burner for seven hours. "My husband won't let me."

I winced. Rosemary was a thorough professional who ruled the Fairfax Hospital ER with an iron fist. None of the ER doctors would dare to cross her. It amused and annoyed me that she could casually tell me that her husband wouldn't let her wear a seat belt.

"Why won't he let you?" I asked incredulously.

"He says it's more dangerous to wear them than not to. He had a friend whose car caught fire and he might have been trapped if he had been seat belted."

"That's possible," I replied, "but it's been clearly proven that in the vast majority of cases, you are much safer wearing a seat belt. You must see it all the time right here in the ER like we do on the ambulance. When you are gambling with your life, doesn't it make more sense to take the better odds?"

Undeterred by logic, Rosemary continued. "Well, what if you drove off a bridge? You wouldn't be able to get out in time if you were wearing a seat belt."

I gave up. Clearly, nothing would convince her to wear a seat belt. And if nothing can convince an emergency room nurse, how is it possible to convince other people? I thought back to the two ambulance calls I had responded to late last August. They had been three days apart.

"Fairfax Police to Fairfax Ambulance."

"Fairfax Ambulance on. Go ahead Fairfax Police."

"An ambulance is needed for a rollover on the northbound lane of the parkway, just north of the Mill Street entrance. The fire department and the state police have been dispatched."

"10–4, Fairfax Police. Ambulance is responding to the northbound lane of the parkway, north of Mill Street, with a crew of two. Please set off the pagers for two more members to meet the ambulance at the scene."

I was at home, finishing some long-delayed letter writing, when I heard the transmission. I grabbed my portable radio and told the police I was responding to the scene. As I bolted out the door, I heard the insistent beep of the pager in my bedroom as the police dispatcher set off the tones in an attempt to get another ambulance corps member to respond.

"45–01 to Fairfax Police," I heard the ambulance call as I sped toward the parkway.

"Go ahead 45–01."

"Be advised we're on location. It looks like a bad one. Advise the helicopter to stand by."

I saw the smoke as I pulled off the parkway behind a volunteer firefighter's car, its blue light flashing on the dashboard. I trotted toward the charred wreckage of what had once been a station wagon, still being hosed down by members of the Fairfax Volunteer Fire Department. Both the front and rear ends of the wagon had been demolished, and the roof had collapsed into the back storage area when the vehicle had rolled over. I was afraid to find out what had happened to the passengers. Had they gotten out before the fire had engulfed the vehicle? Had there been any survivors?

The ambulance was about 50 feet away from the wreckage, but strangely the crew did not seem to be working on any patients. They were talking to a group of people who were watching the firefighters. I ran over to Bob Fiorella.

"Bob," I panted. "How many were there in the car?"

"Four," he replied calmly.

I was baffled by his nonchalance. "Where are they?"

"Right here," he said, motioning toward the man, woman, and two children with whom he had been speaking. "No one seems to be injured."

I stared at the family, incredulously. They certainly appeared to be uninjured. "Are you sure none of you are hurt?" I asked the group.

"Well, I do have this," the man said showing me the back of his left hand.

"Yea," I said, smiling. "That sure is a nasty-looking scratch."

"And I didn't feel it at first, but now my shoulder hurts," the woman said.

"Let me have a look at your shoulder," I suggested.

I pulled her blouse aside and looked at the area of her right collarbone. The woman's skin showed a clear outline of a seat belt.

"Were you all wearing seat belts?" I asked.

They all nodded. "Mommy and Daddy won't drive the car until we all have our seat belts on," the little girl said matter-of-factly.

"Well," I said, gazing at the wreckage of their car. "Your parents are obviously very smart people."

Unfortunately, some people aren't as wise. It was a hot summer afternoon and Sandy McClusky was running late. She needed to finish her shopping before she went to pick up her husband, John, at the airport. He had been away for a week on a business trip, and she wanted to fix a nice dinner tonight. In the backseat, Little John was restless, bouncing from one side to the other.

"God," she muttered, "I can't wait for school to start. If I have to drag him to the store one more time . . ."

"Mommy, Mommy, look what I found on the floor," Johnny yelled from the backseat, leaning forward between the front bucket seats and pulling at her sleeve. Sandy glanced over at her son's hand clutching a grimy penny that had probably been under the front seat for years.

"That's very nice, Johnny, but be a good boy and sit down," she pleaded. "And stay in the center of the seat away from the open windows." Darn busted air conditioner. *When is the garage going to get the part?* she wondered.

Looking into the rearview mirror, she saw Johnny bounce up and down a few times, then turn around and stand on the seat so that he could look out the rear window.

"There's a big truck behind us," Johnny proclaimed. "Vroom, vroom," he shouted, trying to imitate the sound of a truck. He reached down and grabbed his small Tonka truck and ran it back and forth across the ledge below the back window. "Vroom, vroom."

Sandy looked to her left and saw that the mall parking area in front of the supermarket didn't look too crowded. *Maybe it won't take too long*, she thought. Sandy signaled, slowed, and pulled into the left-turn lane of the four-lane road, and waited for an opening in the two lanes of oncoming traffic. The driver of the small gray hatchback that was coming toward her, in the left lane, decided to be "courteous" and stopped to let her make her turn. She waved a thank-you at him and started to pull across in front of the hatchback. She never saw the car that was passing the courteous driver on his right.

I was on duty at headquarters, playing chess with Jack McCaffrey, and losing as usual. But his last move had been a mistake. If he did not become aware of what I was doing, I could mate him in three moves. I reached for my rook. Suddenly the claxon sounded.

No matter how often I hear it, the effect is always the same. All thoughts except the call are instantly forgotten. I felt my heart leap, stimulated by the sound of the raucous horn. I stood, grabbed a pen, and waited by the dispatch pad.

"Fairfax Police to Fairfax Ambulance."

"Fairfax Ambulance on," I said into the mike.

"Respond an ambulance to the entrance to the Mid-County Mall for a 10–2. The time is 14:12."

I quickly jotted down the information and looked at the clock, noting the time of dispatch.

"10–4, FPD. 45–01 is responding to the Mid-County Mall entrance for a personal injury automobile accident."

As I pulled out of the garage, with Jack, the crew chief, riding shotgun and Stephanie DiMartino, our third crew member, in the back, we heard, "Fairfax Police to 45–01."

Jack pulled the microphone off the control panel.

"45–01 on," he yelled over the wail of the siren.

"Our officer at the scene requests that you expedite."

"10–4, FPD."

Expedite: Move your butt, the situation is critical.

As we approached the scene of the accident, I saw a small body lying at the side of the road, a Fairfax officer kneeling over it. Nearby, a young woman appeared to be screaming and was being restrained by bystanders.

I parked the rig, and Jack and I jumped out and went directly to the cop and the patient on the pavement. It was a child, a young boy. His eyes were closed and his face was bluish-gray. The officer was using a resuscitation mask to blow air into the boy's lungs. *Thank God Fairfax cops are trained in CPR,* I thought. Jack took over rescue breathing from the cop while Stephanie ran up with the crash duffel. She pulled out the oxygen cylinder, turned on the valves, and attached a bag-valve-mask.

I went up to the hysterical woman. "What happened?" I asked.

"Help my son!" she screamed.

"What happened?" I yelled again. "Are you all right?"

"I'm fine. Just help him." The woman looked uninjured and was obviously going to be no help with information.

I went back to Stan Poritsky who was now straightening up, rubbing his lower back. His face was filled with an agony that had nothing to do with his back. "What happened?" I asked him.

"The best I can ascertain from witnesses is that, upon impact, the boy was thrown through the car's side window and landed headfirst on the pavement. I checked him out, and he had a pulse but was not breathing, so I started rescue breathing. I don't know much else."

I glanced at the boy's mother, still hysterical.

"The other car?" I asked Stan.

"No one else was hurt." He shook his head. "It wasn't even a serious accident. Not much damage to either car."

I bent over the boy. "He has a pulse, weak and slow," Stephanie said.

"But still no respirations," Jack said. While Jack squeezed the bag-valve-mask, forcing oxygen into the boy's lungs, I quickly examined our patient. The survey usually starts with the top of the head and works downward, but because the boy was being bagged and I wanted Jack to get several full breaths into the boy's lungs, I started at his abdomen and worked upward, looking for blood and feeling for deformity. Abdomen, ribs, neck all felt normal.

I reached around Jack and Stephanie's hands and palpated the boy's skull. I found the problem. The left side of the top of his head was soft where his skull had been crushed. Working around the BVM, I drew up the boy's eyelids to see how his pupils responded to light. The left pupil reacted normally, but the right one remained widely dilated. I turned to Stephanie to ask her to get a child-sized cervical collar and a longboard, but she had anticipated the need and had already put the collar bag and board on the ground beside the crash bag.

We quickly collared the boy and immobilized him on a longboard, then loaded him into the ambulance and sped toward St. Luke's Trauma Center. He coded en route to the hospital, but we were able to restore his pulse with 30 seconds of CPR. He coded again in the ER, and this time, despite the efforts of a medical facility equal to any in the world, his heartbeat could not be restored. He was pronounced dead before we left the hospital.

Passing the scene of the accident on the way back to headquarters, we saw that the car from which the boy had been thrown had not yet been removed. Officer Stan Poritsky was still there, writing out his report. We pulled over to get a better look at the car. The right front end had been damaged, but neither the windshield nor the back window had been broken. The steering wheel was intact, and there had been no invasion of the passenger compartment. The car was probably repairable.

"The boy?" Stan asked us immediately.

I shook my head. "It was just a fender bender," I said, staring at the car. "No one should have been hurt, much less killed."

"No one would have been hurt," Stan replied, "if the mother had obeyed the law and had seat belted her child. Damn! I'd love to prosecute her for vehicular homicide."

Prosecuting her for murder seemed unnecessarily cruel as I remembered the mother's shriek from the hospital waiting room upon being told that her child had died. But maybe, I thought, if just one person buckles his or her child and thus saves that child's life after reading about the prosecution . . .

"Well, it's not our job to make people behave rationally," Jack said from the back of the rig. "We just clean up the mess when they don't."

"Yeah, I know," Stan replied. "And thanks. You guys did a great job."

We got in the rig and slowly, silently rode back to headquarters, each of us immersed in our own thoughts.

○ ○ ○

IT WAS THE beginning of the six-to-midnight shift and Fred Stevens, Joan, and I were checking out the rig. As crew chief, I took the easiest job, holding the clipboard and checking the list while the others called out the contents of each compartment.

Joan was touching each piece of equipment in the large outside compartment. "Stairchair, road flares, shortboard, Kansas Board . . ."

The harsh bray of the claxon vibrated through the ambulance garage. "Fairfax Police to Fairfax Ambulance."

"Fairfax Ambulance on."

"Respond to Hair Event. That's the place next to the diner. We have a report of an explosion with at least one injury at that location. From the report of the caller, expedite."

"10–4, Fairfax Police. Fairfax Ambulance responding to Hair Event, code three."

Fred got into the driver's seat with Joan riding shotgun, and I got into the back. Fred flipped on the master switch while Joan pressed down the bank of red-light indicator switches that activated all of our flashing emergency lights. As we rolled out of headquarters, Fred turned another switch, and the siren began its insistent wail.

We sped down Route 10 toward Hair Event, a beauty parlor in the center of town. I was more anxious than usual. An explosion was a very unusual event for us, and I had no idea what kinds of injuries we would have to deal with.

I took a deep breath to calm myself. I hoped that my hands would not shake as much as they sometimes did on high-pressure calls. It is difficult to appear professionally calm and reassuring when your patient can see that your hands are trembling. He has no way of knowing that the trembling is not from fear or uncertainty, but simply from the large amount of adrenaline that his rescuer's body has produced in response to a possibly life-or-death call.

As we approached Hair Event, we saw that the front window of the beauty parlor was gone. Surprisingly enough, however, there was very little glass on the sidewalk. A crowd of people stood around a black Jeep, parked in front of the salon. I grabbed the crash bag as we rolled to a stop, and sprinted past a policewoman who was talking to several bystanders toward a policeman who was standing next to the Jeep. The acrid smell of gunpowder assaulted me as I got closer to the car.

As I approached, my feet crunched over bits of broken glass and pieces of rubber gasket, probably the remains of the driver's side windows. The windshield was gone and there was extensive damage to the driver's side of the vehicle, but it didn't look like the result of an accident. The metal was bent outward, not bashed in, and, as I got closer I could see that the hood was covered with the remains of the windshield.

"What have you got?" I asked Officer Will McAndrews, who was leaning over the remains of the Jeep.

"The girl in the car is in bad shape."

"What in hell happened?"

"It looks like some kind of explosion in the car. It was powerful enough to demolish the car and blow the front window of the beauty parlor."

"Any injuries in the store?"

"Just some minor cuts and scratches from flying glass. Nobody inside wants medical attention."

"We need the fire department for a wash down," I said, noting the oil and transmission fluid making the asphalt slick.

"They're on the way," Will assured me.

The safety of my crew was my first priority. "Any immediate danger? The car okay? No more explosives?"

"Everything's okay as far as I can tell. Fire department's here just as a precaution."

Just a precaution, I thought. I will brave almost any situation to do my job, but fire is one of my deepest fears. "You sure?"

"Yeah. It's safe enough for you guys to work."

I saw the flashing green light and recognized Jill Tremonte's car. As she pulled to a stop, I yelled to her. "Jill! Check inside the beauty parlor. I'm told everyone's okay, but you'd better make sure." Injuries that seem minor at first often appear much more serious as the body calms down.

I focused on the Jeep. A plain-looking young woman sat behind the wheel, moaning. She appeared to be in her early twenties. Her face was pale, and I could see that she was breathing very rapidly.

"My name is Ed," I said to her. "I'm with the ambulance corps. What's your name?"

Although the woman appeared to be conscious, she did not respond. I saw Joan climb into the passenger side of the Jeep and gently work her way into the backseat.

"I don't think she can hear you," Will said. "The blast may have injured her ears."

"What's your name?" I shouted at her.

"Katya," she cried. "I can't hear you too well."

I found that I had to shout and repeat my questions. "Where are you hurt, Katya?" It was important to establish her responsiveness and level of consciousness.

"My leg. It hurts so bad," she moaned.

"Which leg?" I asked. She looked at me blankly.

"Which leg?" I yelled, moving my mouth closer to her ear.

"My left leg. Please help me."

Most of the side of the car next to her left leg had been blown outward by the blast so that it was not difficult to get at her. Will had a heavy-duty flashlight and shined the light onto the girl's body. Through her partially shredded jeans, I could see that the lower part of her left leg was at an almost right angle to the upper part. There was a considerable amount of blood on what was left of the floor of the car, but the bleeding seemed to have slowed. This wound, at least, was not immediately life threatening.

Before dealing with the leg I needed to check her for other injuries. Sometimes the most obvious injury is not the worst one.

Joan was holding Katya's head stable and talking to her as I quickly used my eyes and hands to survey her body.

"You're doing fine," Joan said loudly. "Try to relax."

"I'm so scared," Katya said. "What's going to happen?"

"We're going to get you out of here as quickly as we can and take you to the hospital so they can give you something for the pain."

"I'm so scared." In spite of the obvious effort it took to talk, Katya's voice was unnaturally loud. I suddenly realized that she could hardly hear her own voice.

"Tell me if anything I do hurts." I said, checking her neck and spine, then her abdomen. No sign of spinal injury.

I placed the diaphragm of my stethoscope just below her left collarbone and said, "Take a deep breath." There were no unusual noises as Katya inhaled. I repeated the procedure on the right side. Her lung sounds were normal.

"Does anything hurt when you breathe?" I yelled.

"No. Just my leg. Help me. It hurts too much. Please help me."

While I was examining my patient, Fred pushed what was probably her pocketbook onto the floor and got into the right side of the car to check her vitals.

"I can't get a radial pulse," he reported. "Her carotid pulse is weak and about one hundred and ten. Her skin is cool and she's diaphoretic." Despite his deliberately calm voice, the news wasn't good. The girl was slipping more deeply into shock, probably from blood loss.

I tried to ignore the sounds of the firefighters laying hose, ready to wet down the engine compartment if anything suddenly caught fire. *God,* I thought, looking at Katya's leg, *sometimes I hate this.*

"Okay, we're going to have to work fast," I replied. I quickly estimated Katya's size and, with Fred's help, fastened an appropriate cervical collar around her neck. "Hand me a pair of heavy shears and then get the MAST."

Fred climbed out of the car, handed me a pair of heavy EMT shears, and went for the antishock trousers. I quickly used the scissors to cut away the denim from Katya's left leg. I was unprepared for the devastation I saw. At a point just below the knee, her leg had been almost completely severed. Only a few strands of skin and connective tissue held the leg together. I swallowed hard and took a breath of air to calm my roiling stomach.

"I can't feel my leg at all now," Katya was saying to Joan. "Is it still there? Please, don't let me lose my leg."

"Try to relax, Katya," I could hear Joan say. "Let us do our job and take the best care of you that we can."

Jill appeared on the passenger side of the car, oxygen cylinder in hand. Functioning as part of the team, she quickly slipped into the passenger seat, put the non-rebreather over Katya's face, and turned up the flow. "Everyone in the store's fine," she said, squeezing Katya's hand. "A few boo-boos but nothing serious." She winked at Katya. More PFA.

I looked at Fred, getting extrication equipment from one of the outside compartments of the rig, pulled the radio out of my back pocket, and keyed the mike. "Fred." As my words echoed from the radio in the rig's cab I saw him turn and look at me. "Bring me every multitrauma dressing you can find and a bottle of sterile saline."

I turned to Katya and Joan. "It's going to hurt like hell when I move your leg," I warned, "but when I'm done, the pain should ease a little." Fortunately there was enough room to manipulate her leg without moving the rest of her body.

Because Joan was just behind Katya's head and she could make Katya hear her, she took charge of psychological first aid. "When we're ready to begin, we're going to count together, good and loud," she said. "By the time we get to sixty, we should be done."

Fred returned within seconds with the MAST, a bottle of sterile saline and an armful of the bulky sterile dressings, the kind that we use for major wounds. When Fred had opened the saline bottle and I had prepared several of the dressings, we were ready to begin. I signaled Joan.

"Okay, Katya, let's count. One, two, three . . ." Loudly, the two women began to count as I moved Katya's severed leg into an approximately "normal" position.

"Sixteen, seventeen . . ."

I placed three 10 by 30s around the injury, wet the dressings with the sterile saline, then used the plastic packaging from the dressings to cover the entire area.

" . . . twenty-one, twenty-two . . ."

It was obvious that Katya was in extreme pain, partly severed nerves sending jumbled messages to her brain. While I held Katya's leg in place, Fred placed additional layers of trauma dressings around the plastic.

" . . . thirty-three, thirty-four . . . We're more than halfway there, Katya," Joan said. "Keep going. Come on. Thirty-five, thirty-six . . ." The two women kept counting.

We used roller gauze to hold the remains of Katya's leg together. While it probably would not save her leg, this temporary reattachment would allow us to put the antishock trousers on her and possibly keep her from dying of shock before we could get her to the hospital. In addition, it was important to try to save as much of her knee as possible. That would allow her to be fitted with an artificial leg more easily, if they couldn't save the limb.

". . . forty-six, forty-seven . . ."

Jill took head stabilization, and we swiveled the girl around and lay her down across the front seat of the Jeep.

". . . fifty-four, fifty-five." Joan heaved a sigh as Katya settled across the seat. "I think the worst is over, Katya. Take a moment to catch your breath."

With her leg bound and no other serious injuries evident, it took only a few moments to slide Katya from the car onto a long backboard and slide the MAST under her. We quickly fastened the Velcro straps of the trousers around her abdomen and legs and attached the pump hoses. I knelt rhythmically on the rubber pump and forced air into the trouser's bladders.

After the MAST was inflated, I was able to feel Katya's radial pulse, and her blood pressure rose to 110 over 70. We quickly strapped her to the backboard, loaded her into the ambulance, and headed for the county trauma center, lights and siren.

"Katya," I said, reaching out to hold her hand. "Tell me a little about yourself."

An only child, Katya had grown up in a small town in Belorussia, at the edge of a birch forest. Life had always been difficult for her and her family. Although she was pretty and intelligent, the future seemed to hold little promise for her. Like so many people of the former Soviet Union, Katya never felt that she could control her own destiny.

Life was poor and regimented, and most of the important personal decisions were made by the state. And Katya had two additional strikes against her: Her parents were not party members, and they were Jewish. She knew that no matter how well she did as a student, she would never be able to go to a university, and that no matter how hard she worked, she would never rise to any level of importance at anything. Chances were that she would not even have a choice of what job she would eventually have.

When Katya's family applied for an exit visa, ostensibly to go to Israel, things became much worse. Her father was immediately fired from his job and they had to live on handouts from a few sympathetic neighbors. The subtle anti-Semitism that they had always felt now became overt.

At school, Katya found that she no longer had any friends. No one would speak to her. And it no longer mattered whether she did her homework or not: Teachers would not call on her, and some even returned her exam papers uncorrected. The only recognition that she got was an occasional muttering of "Jew bitch" from a student who "accidentally" bumped into her or pushed her in the school corridor.

When Katya was thirteen and the family finally obtained permission to emigrate, they left the Soviet Union without a backward glance. They landed in Vienna, the first stop on the trip to Tel Aviv, and breathed the air of freedom. As they had planned, they made some trips to the American embassy. Within a few days they were on their way to Fairfax, where a cousin owned a diner and had offered Katya's father a job.

In America, Katya, basically shy, didn't make friends easily. The teenagers in Fairfax Middle School traveled in cliques with friends they had made years before, groups that excluded all newcomers. As she matured, she didn't blossom as so many girls did. Makeup did little to improve her plain features, and her fine hair didn't lend itself to any of the popular hairstyles. With no dates and few friends, she spent most of her time on her studies.

As a result, she did well in both Fairfax middle and high schools, but, as she progressed, she found it very difficult to make decisions about her future. In Belorussia, there had been no choice of courses. Here, she could choose not only what she would study, but also the level of study. There were general courses, honors courses, advanced-placement courses. There were so many decisions to make.

Deciding about a career was even more daunting. Her grades were good enough to get her into a good college, but she couldn't decide what she wanted to be "when she grew up." She had never had to make such decisions before, and more importantly, she had never felt that she could affect her own future. So Katya decided to take a year off after high school and began to work at the diner as a waitress. That summer she met Joe.

Joe Fortunato was a nice-looking young man about two inches shorter than Katya's five foot six. He had thick, muscular arms from hours of working out and from his heavy work at the car repair shop down the street. He often came into the diner for lunch, still dressed in his coveralls and work boots. He was always alone, and sensing her shyness, he flirted with her the way no one had before. She often caught him looking at her and, although at first it made her uncomfortable, she soon began to meet his eyes. He smiled at her, called her Kathy, and occasionally brought her small presents: a candy bar or a single flower.

One day, while Katya was handing Joe his check, he held her hand, stroking her fingers and making her skin tingle. "Can I see you sometime after work?" he asked. Katya could only nod.

For a few weeks after that, Katya saw Joe almost every evening. At first, he was a sensitive date, easing her along until they were necking in the front seat of his Bronco every evening. Then his attentions became more forceful, and soon he was insisting on doing things that Katya found unpleasant. She began to make up excuses to avoid being with him.

Joe responded to Katya's attempts to distance herself from him by becoming more and more demanding. He would show up at the diner as she finished work and pressure her to go out with him.

One evening, as Katya was leaving the diner, she saw Joe's Bronco in the lot in front of the beauty parlor next to the diner. It was the fourth evening in a row that he had been waiting for her after work, and she decided that this had to end.

"Please, Joe," she said, trying not to sound upset, "just leave me alone."

"Come on, Kathy," he said, using the nickname she had learned to hate, "just a quick hamburger."

"No, Joe. Not tonight."

"Okay. You're just tired. Tomorrow, then?"

Katya shook her head. "I don't think I want to see you again. Please, just go away."

In tears, she turned and walked away, not seeing the rage in Joe's eyes as he watched her leave.

Joe had gone through school in Fairfax four years ahead of Katya. In contrast to Katya, Joe had been the center of attention, negative attention. As the shortest one in the class, he was picked on at every opportunity. In every sport, he was the last selected for the team. When he was twelve, he began lifting weights, but although he developed muscular strength, he never learned how to use that strength to his advantage and he was poorly coordinated. In high school, he was the punching bag for any young man who wanted to take out his frustrations on someone who looked like a formidable opponent but in reality couldn't defend himself.

The army had been just like school in most respects. Joe had made no friends in his unit and was constantly the butt of jokes. But then the army gave him something that was an enormous source of satisfaction to Joe. The army decided to make him a demolitions expert.

Joe had always been a poor student, but now he found that he couldn't learn enough. When he wasn't studying or handling explosives, he would fantasize blowing up all the people who had ever tormented him.

Joe's army training, however, didn't prepare him for a civilian job, so after his discharge he went to work for Jackson's garage in Fairfax. He wasn't a very good mechanic, but the garage owner hired him because he was short of help.

Explosives, however, remained Joe's hobby and his obsession. He turned the basement of his house into a bomb factory, constantly building new devices, which he would detonate in remote areas.

As Joe drove home from the diner and his encounter with Katya, his rage seemed to be a tangible substance—like coal cinders filling his mouth. Everyone had always dumped on him, but this was the ultimate humiliation. He wouldn't take it from that bitch. He knew what to do.

When he got home, Joe went directly down to his basement and assembled the materials that he would need—BBs, gunpowder, and a blasting cap. Then he began to cut a piece of pipe to the proper length.

Katya stepped out of the diner's back door with some trepidation the following evening and was pleased not to find Joe waiting for her. She was looking forward to dinner and a quiet evening at home.

Climbing into the car, Katya threw her pocketbook down on the seat next to her, inserted the key into the ignition, and turned.

As the ambulance raced toward the hospital, Katya alternately complained of intense pain in the severed leg, then of not feeling the leg at all. "I don't want to lose my leg," she pleaded.

"We don't know what's going to happen," Joan said. "We're taking you to St. Luke's where they have specialists who will be able to help you."

"But what will I do if they cut my leg off?"

"You have no choices right now," Joan said, "so worrying about it will get you nowhere. When you have decisions to make, you'll make them."

"They can't cut my leg off. They can't!"

It was all I could do not to say that everything was going to be all right, but I knew she had a long road ahead of her. I had seen the leg and I knew there was little chance of saving it. I could only hope that what

I had done would allow the surgeons to save her knee joint.

"It hurts so much."

Joan reached over, took Katya's hand, and shouted her words of comfort. "Hang on, Katya. Just hang on. When we get you to the hospital, they'll give you something for the pain."

Katya began to cry. "What am I going to do?"

"You can do whatever you have to do. You *will* do whatever you have to."

When we were within radio range of the trauma center, I shouted forward to Fred, "Give me the hospital channel, Fred."

"You got it," he answered, flipping the channel selector on the ambulance radio.

I punched the hospital's code number into the keypad, and when they answered I gave them a brief report on the condition of our patient.

"10-4, Fairfax," the hospital answered. "We'll be expecting you."

Almost three months later, I found a note in my mailbox at the corps. "Dear Joan and Ed. Would you please call me so we can arrange to meet? I'd like to talk with you both. . . ."

The note was signed, "Katya," and then she had written her phone number.

I called and we arranged to meet the next evening at Max's, a local watering hole. We were both surprised as we saw her come through the door. She had a heavy limp, but she was walking.

She saw us immediately and came over. "I wanted you to see me on one of my first nights out," she said as she sat down at our table.

"I'm amazed," I said. "You're doing so well."

"Me, too," Katya said. "I was pretty bad when I first got out of surgery. They told me that the good news was that they had managed to save my knee, thanks to you."

Joan squeezed Katya's hand. "We're so glad."

Katya nodded. "So now I have this artificial beauty," she knocked on her calf, "and I go for physical therapy five times a week. But I'm coming along. I remember what you said in the ambulance, and I guess you were right. I *can* do whatever I have to. And I did."

"That's terrific," I said.

"You heard that they sent Joe up?" Katya asked.

"We read that he had been arrested," Joan said.

"The bastard confessed as soon as they confronted him with the evidence. He'll be in jail for a long time. Forever, I hope." She paused.

"What are you going to do now?" Joan asked.

"The therapy takes up a lot of my time, but I've applied for admission to Fairfax Junior College starting in January. I think I want to study psychology. Learn about people. You know."

"That's great," I said.

"Yeah," she said, "it feels real good. But I still get tired very easily, so I think I'll go home now. My dad's waiting outside in the car." She rose. "The physical therapist says that I'll be able to drive soon." She reached down and tapped her left shin. "No standard shift, though."

"I'm glad you're doing so well," I said. It was amazing how far she had come since the accident, in so many ways.

"Thanks again," she said. "And thank your driver and Jill, too, will you?" She swallowed hard, unable to say more.

"Sure. See you around."

She waved. "See you around."

We get so little feedback; this was especially wonderful.

I learned recently that Joe is now serving his time in the state penitentiary, where he is constantly bullied by the other prisoners.

EPILOGUE

NOW THAT YOU'VE read about us, we hope you have a better understanding of what we do. There are so many stories, one for each of the 1,500 calls the corps responds to each year.

Ed and I like what we do. We like being able to help, and we like working with the members of FVAC, the police and the fire departments. And we like the respect and thanks we get from the people we help.

This morning, Ed and I were standing in line at the diner, waiting to be seated for Sunday breakfast. As we usually do, we were both wearing our navy-blue corps jackets with the star of life on the back and the corps patch on the front.

A nice-looking woman in her fifties passed us on her way out, then turned and asked, "Are you with the ambulance?"

"Yes, I am," I answered proudly.

"I just want to say thank you. You folks are great. You picked me up about two months ago. Not you, but some other of the ambulance people."

"I hope you're feeling better," I said.

"Oh, yes. I guess I had passed out, but I'm better now. They found out I had high blood pressure, and my doctor put me on medicine."

A man whom I assumed to be her husband finished paying their check and walked over. "You guys were so great," he said. "You took care of me, too. I was so scared when I found her lying on the floor."

"Do you remember the date and time?" Ed asked. "I can give your thanks to the crew who picked you up."

"Oh, would you? It was last August twenty-third at about eleven at night.

"Keep up the good work," the man said as he turned to leave.

"And," the woman said, "I'll send a big check to your ambulance corps when I get your fund drive letter."

"Thanks," I said. "Have a good day."

There are thousands of volunteer ambulance corps and rescue squads across the country, all staffed by people like us. If you've ever wanted to help, even in a small way, give the one in your area a call. They all have different facilities, different needs.

Maybe you might like to take an EMT course and help people the way we do, or take CPR or first aid for your own enrichment. Maybe you'd like to dispatch like Greg or become a driver. You might be interested in joining the youth group or the auxiliary.

Whatever you might be able to do, do it. You'll get so much more than you give.

DEFINITIONS OF TERMS

aspirate—draw foreign material into the lungs by inhaling. Aspiration can cause a type of pneumonia that is often fatal.

auscultate—listen to sounds within the body using a stethoscope. The word is usually used when listening for lung or bowel sounds.

backboard—a wooden board approximately six feet long and three feet wide. It is used both as a body splint to support the patient's body and as a lifting aid. Backboards are also called longboards or long spineboards.

BP—blood pressure. BP is an indication of how strongly the heart is beating. Two numbers are usually given (see palp below). The greater number, or systolic pressure, is the pressure when the heart muscle is contracting. The smaller number, or diastolic pressure, is the pressure when the heart muscle is relaxing. Blood pressure might be stated as 120 over 80, meaning 120 systolic and 80 diastolic.

cervical collars—hard-plastic specially shaped bracing devices that surround a patient's neck to prevent additional cervical (neck area) spinal damage.

closed fracture—one in which the skin is not broken.

crash kit—a container, often international orange, that contains emergency supplies for an EMT to use when assisting a patient. The crash kit, often called a crash bag or jump bag, contains such supplies as dressings, bandages, scissors, lights, equipment to take vitals, and gloves. EMTs often carry such a kit in their cars. The crash kit carried in the ambulance, sometimes called a megaduffle, contains oxygen supplies, such as an oxygen cylinder, BVM, oral and nasal airways, and various types of masks, in addition to first-aid equipment.

defibrillator—a machine that can deliver an electrical shock that can jump start a heart that is in V-fib (see below). The defibrillator that we use is semiautomatic. The machine assesses the rhythm and decides whether a shock is indicated. If so, it charges and requests that the EMT-D "press to shock." The manual defibrillator that a paramedic uses merely shows rhythms on a screen and on a tape. From that information, the medic decides which combination of shock, medications, and/or CPR are indicated.

diaphoretic—sweaty.

flail chest—two or more ribs broken in two or more places. The flail segment, the one separated from the remainder of the rib cage, will now move in the opposite direction to the rest of the chest wall causing severe respiratory distress.

Heimlich maneuver—choking maneuver popularized by Henry Heimlich and taught by the American Red Cross and the American Heart Association as part of their CPR courses. For a conscious person who can't talk, breathe, or speak, the Heimlich Hug can dislodge an object obstructing the airway.

jaws of life—gasoline- or electrically powered, hydraulic tool with several attachments that is used to pry metal from around an entrapped patient. The "jaws," also known as the

Hurst Tool, is usually used to disentangle a victim from the automobile around him.

Kling—a brand of roller gauze. Long strips of sterile gauze, prerolled and -packaged, that are used to hold a dressing against a wound. Kling tends to adhere to itself, eliminating the necessity for ties or tape.

logroll—in order to transfer a patient lying on the ground to a backboard, we logroll the patient, turning his body as a unit. This minimizes the possibility of increasing any spinal injury.

normal sinus rhythm—the familiar lub-dub rhythm of the heart. This is the normal rhythm of a functioning heart (See V-fib below).

OB Kit—the obstetrical tools necessary for the emergency delivery of a baby. The kit contains sterile equipment, including gloves, pads, a knife to cut the umbilical cord, and cord clamps.

open fracture—one in which the skin is broken.

palp—short for palpation. Obtaining a blood pressure by palp means that instead of using a stethoscope to listen to the patient's pulse at the inside of the elbow, the patient's radial pulse (see below) is felt while the BP cuff is deflated.

palpate—touch a patient's body with light pressure.

pede-bag—a crash bag containing supplies and equipment in smaller sizes to treat children and infants. In addition, the bag usually contains toys and distractions for younger patients.

pneumothorax—a condition in which air enters the chest cavity, preventing a lung from expanding to draw in air.

point tenderness—indicates that pain is felt when an area of injury is touched or pressed.

pronounce—the process of declaring a patient dead. In most states, EMTs may not pronounce, whereas paramedics may.

pulses—places in the body where an artery runs between a bone and the surface. Pulses can be felt with the fingertips. The radial pulse is found in the wrist, the carotid pulse in the neck, and pedal pulses in various locations in the feet.

Reeves—a Reeves stretcher is a three-foot-wide assembly of six-foot-long plastic slats covered with plastic. A patient can be placed on the Reeves and the unit wrapped around his body. It keeps the spine supported while allowing the patient to be upended or carried at an angle through narrow hallways, over rough terrain, or down stairs. The Reeves has handles at each of the four corners and at the center of each side, permitting a heavy patient to be lifted more easily.

stairchair—a narrow chair with small wheels on the two rear legs and handles for easy carrying. A conscious patient can be seated in the stairchair, belted in, and carried down a flight of stairs or wheeled across a smooth floor.

thoracic—a term that refers to the upper area of the trunk of the body, above the diaphragm and surrounded by the ribs. The thoracic cavity contains the heart and lungs. The thoracic spine connects the ribs in the back.

tib-fib—a short form of tibia-fibula. It refers to the two bones of the lower leg. Because these bones are frequently broken at the same time, a break of the lower leg is referred to as a tib-fib fracture.

turnout gear—coats, pants, hats, and boots made of heavy water- and fireproof material worn by firefighters. We in

FVAC have bright yellow heavy, lined, weatherproof rain and snow jackets that we wear in bad weather.

V-fib—short for ventricular fibrillation. During ventricular fibrillation, the heart's electrical impulses are disorganized and do not cause the heart to beat well enough to circulate blood throughout the body. Unless V-fib is converted to a normal rhythm, possibly by using a defibrillator, the body will die.

vitals—there are several measurable vitals, or vital signs, that indicate the stability of a sick or injured person. The vitals we measure are (1) BP (see above), (2) pulse rate and quality, (3) breathing rate and quality, (4) the appearance, temperature, and moistness of the skin, and (5) the response of the pupils of the eyes to light.

Dear Reader,

Many of you who have just read this book have been involved in situations like the ones described here, either as a rescuer, a patient, or a bystander. We'd love to hear your story and possibly include it, disguised of course, in a future book.

Please write to us:

—Ed Herman and Joan Lloyd
c/o The Publicity Department
The Berkley Publishing Group
200 Madison Avenue
New York, New York 10016